Sociological Insights on Mental Health and Distress

Sociological Insights on Mental Health and Distress

TERESA L. SCHEID, PH.D.
Department of Sociology
The University of North Carolina at Charlotte
Charlotte, NC 28223

S. MEGAN SMITH, PH.D.
Department of Sociology
The University of North Carolina at Charlotte
Charlotte, NC 28223

WILEY Blackwell

Registered Office(s)
John Wiley & Sons, Inc., 111 River Street, Hoboken, NJ 07030, USA
John Wiley & Sons Ltd, New Era House, 8 Oldlands Way, Bognor Regis, West Sussex, PO22 9NQ, UK

For details of our global editorial offices, customer services, and more information about Wiley products visit us at www.wiley.com.

The manufacturer's authorized representative according to the EU General Product Safety Regulation is Wiley-VCH GmbH, Boschstr. 12, 69469 Weinheim, Germany, e-mail: Product_Safety@wiley.com

Library of Congress Cataloging-in-Publication Data

Names: Scheid, Teresa L. author | Smith, S. Megan author | John Wiley & Sons publisher
Title: Sociological insights on mental health and distress / Teresa L. Scheid, Ph.D., Department
    of Sociology, The University of North Carolina at Charlotte [and] S. Megan Smith, Ph.D.,
    Department of Sociology, The University of North Carolina at Charlotte.
Description: Hoboken, NJ : Wiley Blackwell, 2025. | Includes bibliographical references and index.
Identifiers: LCCN 2024056678 (print) | LCCN 2024056679 (ebook) |
    ISBN 9781394200047 paperback | ISBN 9781394200030 epub
Subjects: LCSH: Mental health–Social aspects | Distress (Psychology)–Social aspects | Social psychiatry
Classification: LCC RA790 .S3458 2025 (print) | LCC RA790 (ebook) | DDC 616.89–dc23/
    eng/20250129
LC record available at https://lccn.loc.gov/2024056678
LC ebook record available at https://lccn.loc.gov/2024056679

Cover Image: © agsandrew/Shutterstock
Cover Design: Wiley

Set in 10/12 pts STIXTwo by Lumina Datamatics

To Virginia Aldige Hiday. Thank you for introducing me to the sociological study of mental health, your mentorship and colleagueship, and to your continued friendship. Teresa L. Scheid.

To my parents, whose consistent and unwavering support propels my passion to educate, raise awareness, and reduce stigma around mental health. Thank you for standing alongside me during all the obstacles and challenges over the years that have become stepping stones. Megan Smith.

Contents

Part 2   Unpacking the Relationships Between Stress, Social Supports, and Mental Health   47

Part 3   Structural Sources of Mental Distress   101

Part 4   The Complexities of Care   149

Preface

Sociological Insights on Mental Health and Distress provides a readable, accessible, undergraduate-level textbook which seeks to help students understand the important role that social factors play in understanding mental health and distress. Mental distress is both a personal trouble and a public issue to use terms introduced by C. Wright Mills in his 1959 book *The Sociological Imagination*. Mills argued that our individual problems must be understood within the context of a given society, within a given historical period. We utilize the larger conceptual framework of the Sociological Imagination, examining the connections between the individual experience of mental health problems, the social and structural sources of mental health issues, and the larger cultural and historical context. Our goal is to introduce a wide range of students to the insights sociologists offer into the social sources of our mental health problems.

The authors, Scheid and Smith, have an extensive record of scholarship and teaching and collaborated on an earlier book *Ties That Enable: Community Solidarity for People Living with Serious Mental Health Problems*, published by Rutgers University Press in 2021. *Ties That Enable* built upon our extensive research in the development of community-based solutions to the problems faced by people living with severe mental health problems. *Sociological Insights* is oriented to a much broader range of readers who share an interest in mental health, including students and providers in psychology, public health, and social work. Dr. Scheid assumed responsibility for the writing of the text, drawing on over 30 years as a mental health scholar and teaching upper-level and graduate-level courses in the Sociology of Mental Health and Illness. Her PowerPoint lectures are available through the ancillary website for the text. She has been co-editor of three editions (1999, 2010, 2017) of *A Handbook for the Study of Mental Health: Social Contexts, Theories, and Systems* and a substantial revised 4th edition (*Sociology of Mental Health: Theories, Contexts and Systems*) will be available in 2025 (Cambridge University Press). Dr. Smith has extensive experience and training in newer pedagogical techniques and has developed introductory courses in mental health. She assisted with the development of the textbook and provided extensive feedback on each chapter. She assumed primary responsibility for additional teaching materials and resources to accompany the text which are available via the website. Both authors share a commitment to writing intensive courses and reflective writing as well as the use of readings that combine classic insights with current research. In addition to research and teaching, we devote considerable time to working with local mental health agencies and stakeholders to improve mental health. Our goal is to have students read and think about the many complexities of mental health we describe; to this end, the text is short. concise and accessible. Our voice is active, first person and conversational, and we avoid the extensive use of references. Learning resources and student activities are geared toward reflection, active learning and applications, with a focus on lived experience and examination of data. We end the book with considerations for social change, asking "what would a mentally healthy society look like?"

Acknowledgements

First and foremost, we need to acknowledge the role of the classic and contemporary theorists which have shaped our own understandings of mental health, as well as the wider field of the Sociology of Mental Health: Emile Durkheim, Erving Goffman, and Allan Horwitz. We also want to acknowledge each other and our mutual appreciation for classical and contemporary theory. We have continued to share our understandings of mental health and distress in our continued advocacy, research and teaching. Our students have also contributed to our evolving understanding of the mental health crisis for young people. Students in Dr. Scheid's undergraduate and graduate classes in mental health provided useful feedback on "Sociological Insights" throughout 2023 and 2024. Dr. Smith piloted many of the accompanying teaching resources (available via a web page) in her introductory mental health class. We want to thank the external reviewers who made detailed comments and helped us to improve the book. Also, many thanks to the Wiley editors and production staff who brought this book to publication.

List of Abbreviations

ADHD: Attention Deficit Hyperactivity Disorder

BIPOC: Black, Indigenous, People of Color

CDC: Centers for Disease Control and Prevention

DSM: Diagnostic and Statistical Manual

LGBTQ+: Lesbian, Gay, Bisexual, Trans, Queer

MHP: Mental Health Problems

NHIS: National Health Interview Survey

NIMH: National Institutes of Health

PSMH: People with Severe Mental Health Problems

PTSD: Post-traumatic Stress Disorder

SAMHSA: Substance Abuse and Mental Health Services
Administration

SES: Socioeconomic Status

WHO: World Health Organization

Introduction

Mental health has become front-page news with continued public attention to what is referred to as the mental health crisis. Young people are especially vulnerable; they have experienced online learning, social isolation, family stressors, and difficulties establishing meaningful social relationships. The dramatic increases in levels of anxiety, depression, loneliness, and suicide have been well-documented. Suicide is the major cause of death for young people worldwide. How can we make sense of the global mental health crisis? In describing *The Sociological Imagination*, C. Wright Mills (1959:10) noted that "many public issues are described as psychiatric; often it seems in a pathetic attempt to avoid the larger issues and problems of modern society." How true today! The problem is that we focus on personal troubles (for example, incidences of suicide) and fail to address the structural sources of our individual problems, those social factors that may account for rising rates of suicide among younger people. Sociology provides insights into how larger social forces have affected our mental health. Specifically, the mental health crisis is a result of rapid social change, structural strains, and social inequality. The insights offered by sociology not only help us make sense of our experiences but also empower us to take control of our mental health and to create a social environment that promotes positive mental health. Rather than describing the wide range of theoretical perspectives developed by sociologists, we identify four key concepts that distinguish what sociology has to offer to our understanding of mental health from the more common biological or psychological perspectives that focus on the individual. These concepts are as follows.

1. Context: Sociologists focus on the social context within which mental health problems are defined, experienced, and treated. In social context, sociologists refer to the social structures (including groups, organizations, institutions, economic and political systems, and cultures) as well as the values and beliefs that shape these social structures. While mental illness is experienced as a personal trouble, it is a public issue requiring social solutions. Sociologists focus on mental health and illness in its social context, as opposed to the biological and psychological approaches that reduce mental health problems (MHPs) to individual pathology.

2. Integration: From Emile Durkheim (one of the founding fathers of sociology) to contemporary research on social relationships, our connection to others is the primary source of mental health. Social integration refers broadly to our ties to each other, our social bonds, and degree of group cohesion. Our family, friends, peers, significant others, and extended social networks all have a major impact on our social relationships and social supports, which play a critical role in our mental health.

3. Stress: Structural strains (such as unemployment) produce stress. While we all experience stress, sociologists understand that stress is unequally distributed, with those in the lower status positions experiencing higher levels of chronic strains. COVID-19 was a major stressor that exacerbated existing inequalities with minority groups experiencing higher rates of illness, unemployment, and mental distress, and we devote considerable attention to COVID-19 throughout the text. In addition to gender, age, race, and ethnicity, our social roles and identities are important sources of social status and position and vulnerability to stress.

4. Stigma: There has always been a great deal of stigma associated with MHPs. A stigma is an attribute that is discrediting and involves stereotypes that can result in active discrimination. There is a long and important sociological tradition that has advanced our understanding of both the sources and consequences of the stigma surrounding MHPs. Stigma resistance is an important sociological advance to the understanding of stigma and how to combat it.

These four sociological insights operate synergistically and do not comprise discrete "topics." Instead, they all contribute to the sociological understanding of mental health and MHPs. Each chapter in this book examines how these sociological insights shape mental health and distress. We utilize a scaffolding approach where these core concepts are introduced in early chapters, and then further developed and applied in later chapters. There is a focus throughout this book on youth mental health, which was listed as a top priority for both the World Health Organization and the United States White House in 2022. There are also global initiatives addressing youth mental health, including the World Health Organization and the Global Alliance for Behavioral Health and Social Justice. In the United States, Mental Health America has been central in providing resources for youth advocacy and peer supports, as well as addressing suicide prevention and school-based reforms.

The book is organized into four parts, each with three chapters. An introduction to each part provides more specific information on the topics we will cover. The parts are organized within the more common framework articulated by C.W. Mills as the "Sociological Imagination" where individual issues must be understood within the context of a given society as social problems, which are shaped by the wider cultural and historical framework. The *Sociological Imagination* has been usefully applied to our understanding of health and illness (Hinote and Wasserman, 2020). In addition, we address issues related to cultural variability. Repeatedly throughout the book, we make reference to the important difference between individualist and communal cultures, which shapes the societal response to mental health and distress.

In Part I, we start at the individual level and discuss what it means to have an MHP. Are you mentally ill, abnormal, deviant, mad, depressed, anxious, or suicidal? Are MHPs disabilities? A key distinction is between the "worried well" (all of us have MHPs at one time or another) and those with more severe and persistent MHPs. Sociologists are generally critical of reductionist approaches and assessment tools that assume you are either mentally well or ill, as well as the over-reliance on medical approaches to treatment of MHPs. Instead, many sociologists focus on degrees of wellness or distress, flourishing or languishing. We also introduce ideas about medicalization and neurodiversity. We then turn to an extended discussion of anxiety as a widely shared mental health issue that can be seen as a normal response to stress and uncertainty.

In Part II, we consider aspects of our social structure that directly influence our mental health: stress and social relationships. We all experience stress, though the sources of stress have changed. It is the inability to control stress as well as our response to stress, which produces mental distress. The stress process model posits that social context and status inequalities produce stress, which place some groups at greater risk for MHPs. We use COVID-19 to illustrate what is referred to as the stress process model. Social supports provide ways to cope with stress and thus can help buffer the effects of stress on mental health. While generally seen as a source of social support, group membership can also increase an individual's vulnerability to stress. An individual's sense of "self" is important to responses to stress and is shaped by social context as well as relationships with others and our social roles. We therefore provide a brief description of identity theory and its relevance to understanding the discredited identity associated with MHPs. We also address the college environment as an important social context for stress and social support, as well as mental distress. We included the sociological approach to understanding suicide in Part II given high rates of suicide among college students. Sociological theories about suicide focus on social integration as well as social conflict. We describe recent research on the role of social contagion in influencing suicide rates and we provide guidelines for suicide prevention efforts.

In Part III, we turn to the broader structural sources of mental health and distress. Key to understanding the wider social context of mental health is social stratification, which is the primary source of inequality, intersectionality, and stigma. Stigma serves as a major barrier to treatment and mental health care. Individuals may delay seeking care for fear of being labeled; families and communities are reluctant to acknowledge MHPs, and societal-level stigma reduces public support for programs that can provide mental health care and social supports. Homelessness is a consequence of the marginalization experienced by those with serious MHPs and economic dislocation, so we spend some time discussing the reality of homelessness for those with serious MHPs. Individuals with other discredited identities, including racial minorities, and individuals experiencing gender diversity are also marginalized and subsequently have higher levels of mental distress. We draw attention to the experience of homelessness for LGBTQ+ youth. The stigma surrounding mental health intersects with other marginalized social status positions, and we address ideas about stigma resistance.

In Part IV, we move the wider societal framework within which mental health care operates, addressing approaches to treatment and care and changing values and priorities. Mental health care is complex, with a variety of different types of patients, professional groups who provide care, and diverse systems of care. In addition, financing mental health care is confusing and inadequate. We describe the various historical cycles of mental health care and address whether the focus has been on care or social control. The lack of support for resources for community integration is certainly a major source of our global mental health crisis. Involuntary outpatient commitment can be seen as a form of benevolent coercion, with reference to assisted treatment emphasizing therapeutic care. A major issue is the right to refuse treatment, including medications. At its most extreme social control is evident in the criminalization of those with serious MHPs.

In our mental health classes (both in person and online), we have found that the use of documentaries is an excellent resource for helping readers to visualize the social sources and consequences of mental health and distress. Reading is a rational activity, while visualization is more emotional. Combing reading with visualization leads to a more complete understanding of mental health and distress. Throughout the book, we will make suggestions for documentaries or movies to accompany the students' reading. An excellent introduction for students and the public is the PBS series *The Mysteries of Mental Illness*, which aired in 2021. The four-part documentary uses historical evidence, interviews, and personal accounts to provide a comprehensive account of the ways in which social conditions have shaped our understanding of mental health and distress. In Appendix A, we provide a brief summary of the documentary and include discussion questions related to the documentary throughout the text. We encourage readers to view the documentary to enhance their understanding of the many issues we describe and discuss in this book.

In addition, we utilize primary readings in our classes and highly recommend Robert Kolker's 2021 book, *Hidden Valley Road: Inside the Mind of an American Family* (Anchor Books). The book does an excellent job of addressing the major theories, treatments, and understandings of mental illness as well as a very readable review of the scholarship that is critical of psychiatric research. Kolker's account also documents not only how treatment changed over time but also how the stigma of mental illness changed. Rather than an academic text, the book follows a journalistic approach and is as compelling to read as any mystery novel. At the same time, the depth and breadth of the information provided by Kolker meets the standards of a rigorous scholarship, but presented in an engaging manner. A brief summary is provided in Appendix B.

Dr. Scheid augments student reading of *Hidden Valley Road* with Owen Whooley's 2019 historical account of psychiatry (*On the Heels of Ignorance: Psychiatry and the Politics of Not Knowing*, University of Chicago Press). Whooley argues that madness may not be knowable, and that its incomprehensibility terrifies us (p. 220). By viewing mental illness as a disease (or the product of faulty wiring), "psychiatry allows us the luxury of recoiling from the raving delusions of the schizophrenic, the cheerless gloom of the depressed, the nervous jittering of the anxious, and the tumultuous mood swings of the manic." How do we cope? Avoidance, compassion, fatigue, and stigmatization, with little support for community-based systems of care, leaving those with serious MHPs to fend for themselves in jails or on the streets. As Whooley eloquently states (p. 222), "A 'non-system' as callous and ineffective as this can only exist when supported by a deep and abiding indifference to those that we force to endure it."

We hope that *Sociological Insights* challenges its readers to be less complicit and to work toward reforms within their communities. In the final chapter, we utilize the WHO 2022 *World Mental Health Report: Transforming Mental Health for All*, to provide a vision for the future and concrete strategies that we hope will empower students. We draw upon the framework for mental health reform and justice we introduced in our 2021 book, *Ties That Enable*, to illustrate that reform must be both top down and bottom up. Social structures can enable individuals, but individuals must also exercise their agency to change the social structures that surround them. The potential for major social change is the promise of the "Sociological Imagination." How can social structures be reformed so as to empower individuals? What kinds of social structures are needed to promote mental health? How can social systems promote equity and social justice? We agree with the WHO that community-based advocacy and stigma resistance are two critical strategies, which can build upon the lived experiences of individuals and which students and readers can engage in.

References

Hinote, B.P. and Wasserman, J.A. (2020). *Social and Behavioral Science for Health Professionals*, 2e (ed. Lantham, Maryland): Rowman & Littlefield.

Mills, C. W. (1959). *Sociological Imagination*. New York: Oxford University Press.

Scheid, T.L. and Smith, S.M. (2021). *Ties That Enable: Community Solidarity for People Living with Serious Mental Health Problems*. New Brunswick, NJ: Rutgers University Press.

Whooley, O. (2019). *On the Heels of Ignorance: Psychiatry and the Politics of Not Knowing*. Chicago, IL: University of Chicago Press.

PART 1

Understanding Mental Health Problems

What does it mean to have a mental health problem? Are you mentally ill, abnormal, deviant, or distressed? Are mental health problems illnesses, disorders, or disabilities? A key distinction is between the "worried well" (all of us have mental health problems at one time or another) and those with severe persistent mental health problems. In Chapter 1, we address the definitions and cultural understandings of mental health problems. A distinction is made between the medical model and the disability model of mental health problems, and sociological theories about labeling and medicalization are introduced. In Chapter 2, we examine various theories about the causes or sources of mental health problems. We contrast psychological, biomedical, and sociological approaches, and introduce the biopsychosocial model. Central to debates over the sources of mental health problems are whether symptoms are culturally dependent or not. If universal, i.e. symptoms of a given disorder are the same across cultural contexts, there is arguably an underlying biological source. If there is evidence of cultural variability, mental health and distress can be seen as being shaped by cultural and social definitions as to what is "normal" versus "abnormal" behaviors. This leads to a discussion of labeling theory, which views psychiatric symptoms as violations of social norms rather than inherent pathologies. In Chapter 3, we address issues related to the assessment of mental health problems, i.e. how do we determine whether a person has a mental health problem? Further, how do researchers determine how many people in the population have mental health problems? Some may think of this as a diagnosis, but this assumes a categorical understanding whether you either have a mental health condition or you do not. Many sociologists are critical of reductionist approaches and assessment tools, which assume you are either mentally well or unwell. Instead, clinicians and researchers need to assess degrees of wellness or distress along a continuum. Chapter 3 ends with an extended discussion of anxiety to illustrate the issues related to assessment of mental health and points to the role that social factors play in variations of mental health problems.

Learning Resources

Readers and students are encouraged to view the first two episodes of the Ken Burns documentary *Hiding in Plain Sight: Youth Mental Illness* (released in 2022 and available through PBS). The documentary provides insight into the lives of a diverse group of 20 young people who describe their experiences of mental health and distress. A student in one of Dr. Scheid's mental health classes felt: "It was extremely validating to hear other people share their experiences and have an array of reasons for why people have mental health problems... Something that may seem insignificant to one person, may be the source of trauma for another. Not only is it different for every person, but for some people, it may even be different every day. This can make it difficult for someone to fully understand their mental health on their own, much less to try to explain it to someone else. Similarly, many people are conditioned to think that they have to manage their own mental health and that they shouldn't reach out to other people about it. To quote the documentary, 'The first, and often most difficult step, is to simply start talking about it'. This hit me hard, but it's extremely true. I find the most difficult part about trying to reach out is the fear of the unknown."

For discussion: What insights did the video provide to you about the experience of mental distress?

CHAPTER 1

What Does It Mean to Have a Mental Health Problem?

While in the past mental health problems (MHPs) were relegated to the attic, or in some cases the closet, we are now confronted by the "mental health crisis" with increased rates of depression, anxiety, and suicide. What does it mean to have an MHP? Are you mentally ill, abnormal, deviant, or mad? Are you depressed, anxious, suicidal, or just sad? Are you dangerous, out of control, a threat to society, or bad? Are you neurotic or psychotic? Are MHPs disabilities? Are you doing as well as you can, or are you struggling to get by? While all of us will experience MHPs at one time or another, many people live with severe and persistent MHPs. It is important to differentiate between MHPs, which are acute, or short-term, and chronic long-term conditions. Mechanic (2006) provided a useful distinction that positioned individuals with MHPs into three groups. The first group are those with typical mental health issues such as normal depression following a loss or some other stressful event. The second group are those with acute MHPs that are more severe, or those with chronic conditions but who also can maintain normal role functions. The third group are those with serious, chronic mental conditions that involve significant functional disability, the largest group of which are those diagnosed with schizophrenia or psychosis. In this chapter, we address the definitions and cultural understandings of MHPs.

Defining Mental Health and MHPs

Mental health was not formally defined until 1961, despite the existence of the National Institute of Mental Health, which had an annual budget of US$91 million. At that time, Dr. William Menniger defined mental health as:

> *"The adjustment of human beings to the world and each other with a maximum of effectiveness and happiness. Not just efficiency, or contentment, or the grace of obeying the rules of the game cheerfully. It is all of these together. It is the ability to maintain an even temper, an alert intelligence, socially considered behavior, and a happy disposition. This, I think, is a healthy mind."*

While this definition of mental health clearly raises some concerns over compliancy in a world gone array (with the threat of nuclear war facing Americans in the early 1960s and once again today), the current definition of mental health also emphasizes a certain calm acceptance of the social world. The World Health Organization (WHO 2022) defined mental health as "a state of mental well-being that enables people to cope with the stressors of life, to realize their capabilities, to learn and work well, and to contribute to their communities" (World Health Organization [WHO 2022]; Box 1.1). Coping is important, but equally important is challenging, empowerment, or advocacy – efforts to change those social structures that contribute to poor mental health.

The WHO definition of mental health emphasizes that mental health is not merely the absence of a mental disease. Instead, then and now, mental health involves an understanding of well-being or positive mental health. The aspects of "positive" mental health include:

1. Self-esteem: The attitude the individual has toward themselves.
2. Self-actualization: The degree the individual realizes their potential through actions.
3. Coherence: Unification of aspects of the individual's personality or sense of self.
4. Autonomy: A degree of independence from social influences.
5. Mastery: The ability to take life as it is and move forward.

We draw on Ryff (1985) to provide a deeper understanding of the components of well-being. We begin with self-esteem, which is not only what we might think about having a high sense of personal value or importance, but fundamentally involves self-acceptance. Do you know your strengths and limitations? Do you have a coherent sense of self that accepts both good and bad qualities? Do you have a positive sense of your past, or have you been able to place negative events into a coherent framework or explanation that leads to acceptance? Self-acceptance is critical to positive social relations with others. Positive interactions are based on trust, the capacity for empathy, concern about others, and an understanding of the give and take of human interaction. Social relationships involve not only intimacy and affection but also autonomy and independence. Adolescence is a time when young people move from compliance with authority to greater independence. Learning to resist social pressures, rather than conformity, is critical to mental health. Autonomy builds upon the ability to regulate your own behavior and to follow your own standards, and not simply follow the crowd. Can you think of examples from your own experience growing up where you faced pressures to conform?

The final component of positive mental health, and one which we refer to often in this book, is mastery. Mastery has to do with control, defined as the ability to cope with environmental demands, and is critical to being able to deal with the many sources of stress we face in life. Critical to mastery is knowing your own capabilities and then selecting or creating those situations which allow you to succeed. A very common example is your choice of major. Maybe you always wanted to be a doctor. Your mother may have been a doctor, or you had a great experience with a doctor as a child. You then enrolled in the prerequisite biology and chemistry courses and failed miserably. However, you really liked your health class and elected to pursue a different major, maybe Psychology, Public Health, Social Work, or Sociology. Mastery is closely related to having realistic aims and objectives for yourself. A sense of purpose will contribute to continued personal growth and development, as well as openness to new experiences, all of which are critical to positive mental health over the life course. Unfortunately, we spend far too little time talking about mental health and instead focus on our MHPs.

In recent years, MHPs have been viewed as diseases to be diagnosed and treated, reflecting a medical approach to mental health. Diagnoses are based on symptoms, with medical treatment providing for the management of these symptoms. Treatment involves medication or other types of medical intervention such as electric shock therapy with less reliance on psychosocial therapy. Sociologists are generally critical of individualist models that reduce MHPs to a disease or genetic explanation, instead placing greater emphasis on the social environment or context of the MHP. Unemployment, discrimination, isolation, conflict, poverty, and inequality are all structural strains that have negative impacts on health and well-being. Furthermore, social and environmental contexts influence the individual's self-concept, relations with others, autonomy, and mastery, which also have major impacts on our mental health. We turn to a consideration of the WHO definitions of mental distress, which is used to provide global estimates of mental health.

While the WHO (2022) does not define mental health issues as simply the absence of disease, they do rely on the International Classification of Diseases (ICD-11), to define mental disorders as "clinically significant disturbances in an individual's cognition, emotional regulation, or behavior that results in dysfunction." Dysfunction is defined to refer to distress or impairment in important areas of functioning, which is a broad category that includes our social, family, school, occupational, or any other area of life. While not clearly stated, the WHO emphasis on dysfunction implies there is a "normal" level of functioning: that you can get up, get dressed, go to school or work, and meet the normative obligations of social life.

The term psychosocial disability is used by the WHO (2022) to refer to long-term disabilities, which interact with structural barriers (such as stigma) that limit the ability of an individual to participate equally in meeting normative expectations. Finally, a mental health condition is a very broad term that refers to any disorder, disability, or any other mental health issue that produces distress or disability. The WHO definition of a mental health condition reflects the original formulation of a mental disorder codified in the Diagnostic and Statistical Manual, which states that a mental disorder causes distress and impaired functioning. The WHO has replaced the term "disorder" with "condition" – most likely as an effort to avoid stigmatization. Whether a disorder or a condition, MHPs (the term we use most often) are not seen as normal. But perhaps they are normal? Sadness is normal; anger is normal; anxiety is normal. Sociologists have argued that what are viewed as MHPs are often normal responses to our social environment.

Depression provides a good example of normal versus abnormal responses to life events. We have all experienced some degree of depression, when a loved one died or a relationship ended, feeling not only sad but also unable to meet our normal obligations, such as going to class or work. Sleeping or eating too little or too much, binge-watching Netflix, and avoiding normal activities are all typical responses to loss. But grief and sadness are part of everyday life; it is when we are depressed and unable to function for no good reason that we need to seek out additional care and support. The important distinction is that we all feel distressed at times, but when there is no apparent source for our distress, then we may have a mental health condition that needs attention.

Consider anxiety, which we all experience at different times throughout our lives. Rates of anxiety have been increasing in the past two decades, with anxiety becoming the most widely experienced mental health condition. Almost everyone has had high levels of anxiety due to not only COVID-19, but concerns over political polarization, racial injustice, and climate change. We also have anxiety over our mental and physical health, newly termed as health anxiety. Simply meeting the everyday demands of relationships, family, school, and future aspirations can all produce anxiety. While anxiety is a "normal" state given the many demands we face throughout the life course, our mental health is enhanced by learning how to cope with these demands and to develop a sense of mastery, or control. We all remember the anxiety we felt over our first performance, be it an in-class presentation, dance or music recital, sporting event, or entrance exam for college. If we failed to live up to expectations (both our own and those of others) hopefully, we tried again and learned and did better the next time. Failure is essential to learning and mastery, as it forces us to challenge ourselves and to grow. The essence of mental health is developing the skills to cope with many demands life will throw at us. For those facing insurmountable obstacles, such as poverty or abuse, resilience is an important aspect of mental health.

When we are unable to meet the demands placed upon us, we may experience an impairment or dysfunction. Rather than trying to do our best, some may retreat and not go to school, or work, or attend social functions. The anxiety may be overwhelming, causing difficulties in sleeping, eating, or even figuring out what to wear. Depression is also a likely consequence, with the loss of self-worth when you fail to meet the expectations you have set for yourself. You may seek medical care and be diagnosed with generalized anxiety disorder, depression, or another clinical condition. Hopefully, recognition of the problem and its source (see Chapter 2) results in some kind of intervention where you learn effective coping skills to deal your mental health issues. For many, exercise, eating well, and maintaining a regular schedule, as well as seeking out social supports all work to enable us to deal with many MHPs. In addition to these sources of positive mental health, some people may need therapy and others may need medication.

If the difficulty an individual faces is long-term and they are not able to meet social expectations, the disorder meets the conditions of a disability. Serious MHPs (for example, schizophrenia) often meet the criteria of a disability because the individual cannot fulfill what are considered normative (i.e. socially defined) expectations, such as holding a job. In addition to the persistent nature of the disorder, the stigma associated with more serious MHPs is apparent when communities are not accepting of those who violate what are seen as normal behaviors. Someone who talks out loud to the voices in their head, or has trouble maintaining meaningful social interactions, will also have trouble holding onto a job and will need more community support, not less.

MHPs as Disability

The sociological emphasis on the social context of mental health and illness can be framed within a disability model, rather than the medical model that pathologizes individual behaviors. The disability model of mental health links disability to relationships and structures in society, rather than to the individual. Disability is not just a matter of individual health or psychiatric symptoms, rather how the roots of disability lie in society. Disabilities are made worse by society's inability to either provide or create supportive environments. With a medical model, emphasis is placed on diagnosis, treatment, and cure of individuals. Under a disability model, there is recognition that MHPs often involve long-term impairment and loss of functioning – no matter what the "cause" of the disability may be. Responsibility for treatment is placed on the social structures that marginalize and exclude those who are seen as different, or who do not fit the criteria for inclusion. Just as sexism excludes women from positions of power, "ableism" excludes those seen as disabled.

With physical disabilities, we have learned to build ramps or provide other needed accommodations, but the accommodations for MHPs are less clear and may involve interactions with other people, such as with a supervisor at work.

A view of MHPs as disabilities is firmly grounded in a social model of health and points to the importance of modifying social structures to promote the capacities and strengths of individuals, ideals that have been emphasized by the movement to recovery. Recovery seeks to provide those living with disabilities a meaningful place in society and a sense of wellness. Viewing mental illness as a disability expands the focus for "treatment" to the wider society and the social sources of institutionalized oppression, which includes the stigma of being labeled as mentally ill or disabled. However, the "label" matters and Mulvany (2008) described controversy within disability theory over differences between different types of disabilities and whether the term "impairment" should be used to refer to the unique challenges of "disorganized thinking." MHPs raise important questions as to what accommodations are needed to help an individual in school or at work.

Psychosocial rehabilitation builds on a view of MHPs within a disability framework, with the goal to improve the capacity of individuals with disabling MHPs to "function" well in society and to fulfill normal role expectations, with an emphasis on work. However, the focus is on building upon the adaptive competencies or capabilities of the individual, rather than in changing social structures to allow for a sense of accomplishment despite having an MHP. The disability framework is critical for those who experience long-term, serious, or persistent MHPs such as schizophrenia. Schizophrenia has a long history pointing to incomprehensible actions and behaviors characterized by delusions, hallucinations, hearing voices, and the experience of an alternative reality. These spells of psychotic behavior are often episodic, meaning that there will be relatively stable periods that still involve MHPs, including a high vulnerability to stress, difficulty with interpersonal relationships, poor coping skills, and many other functional limitations including learning. However, a psychotic episode or break can occur with little advance warning or explanation. Given the lack of coherence, or evidence of a reality deficit, those who are "mad" are often seen as bad or as threatening and in need of social control or confinement. Disability theorists are generally critical of efforts to control an individual, seeing the root of illness as lying in society.

MHPs as Violations of Social Norms

Those with more serious MHPs generally exhibit what we view as abnormal or inappropriate behavior, such as talking or laughing out loud when no one else is there. Such behaviors lie outside common social norms, and consequently a deviance perspective has been used by many sociologists to understand MHPs. In a classic formulation, Scheff (1984, p. 40) argued that "psychiatric symptoms such as withdrawal, hallucinations, continual muttering, or posturing may be categorized as violations of certain social norms. There norms are so taken for granted that they are not explicitly verbalized." Sociologists understand that what counts for "normal" is based upon widely accepted definitions of what is acceptable. These definitions are socially constructed; that is, we interpret behavior and actions within a given social context as to what is "normal" depending on our social expectations. These cultural beliefs about normative, or acceptable, standards are often reflected in psychiatric definitions of mental health disorders. In the past, homosexuality and premenstrual syndrome were classified as psychiatric disorders, and we see current debates over gender identity as an abnormal behavior. We will return to these debates for psychiatric classification of disorder in the following chapters, but an important issue is how we make determinations as to what is normal and what is not, or who is sane and who is insane. These decisions about what is "normal" are based on our definition of the situation; is the individual following the rules of appropriate behavior for a given social context? Behavior that might seem odd in one context could be quite normal in another.

What is important about the label of "mentally ill" is that it overrides all other definitions of the situation, and that even normal behavior can provide evidence of abnormality (Goffman, 1961). As seen in the popular movie "One Flew Over the Cuckoo's Nest" and reflected in Rosenhan's (1973) study of pseudo-patients admitted to psychiatric hospitals, views of sanity and insanity are socially constructed and reflect the prevailing definition of the patient as either mentally ill or not. The movie reflects the finding of Rosenhan that psychiatrists and medical personal often cannot detect that their patients are in fact "normal," although fellow patients quickly recognized that the pseudo-patients were not in fact "mentally ill." While Rosenhan's pseudo-patients all described their "normal" life histories and relationships, their histories were interpreted as reflecting abnormal behaviors. All but one of the patients was subsequently released as "schizophrenic in remission," indicating that "sanity" was never recognized, according to individuals, initially defined to be "insane."

While there has been some criticism of Rosenhan's study based on concerns over the credibility of his data (Scull 2023), the important point is that a diagnosis does not reside within an individual but is shaped by the context within which the behavior occurs. Slater (2004) decided to recreate Rosenhan's study by seeking treatment for the same symptoms used in the original study; hearing voices that said "thud." Slater is interesting as she herself was institutionalized in 1976 "for doing things fourteen-year-olds do and then some" (p. 74). She describes the "bin," as she calls it, with the kids trading "diagnoses like marbles," but she got sicker in the hospital and began cutting herself. In repeating the experiment, Slater, now a wife, parent, psychologist, and successful author, went to nine different emergency rooms and while she was never admitted to the hospital, she was released with a diagnosis of depression with psychotic features and given a combination of anti-psychotic and antidepressant medications. It is important to note that she reported that she was sleeping well, eating well, and not experiencing any stress, but she was a bit bothered by hearing the voice saying "thud." It is also important to note that while her visits with psychiatrists were short (around 10 minutes), they were all very nice to her. Slater (2004, p. 75) concluded that there is "some essential truth in Rosenhan's findings. Labels do determine how we view what we view."

While processes of social construction are clearly important to understanding the identification of "abnormal" behavior, a more fundamental process involves the way we all label some behaviors as "incomprehensible" and then conclude there is a serious MHP at the root of the behavior we cannot understand. Horwitz (1982) argued that the less sense a behavior or action makes to us, that is – how incomprehensible it is – the more likely we are to label the person exhibiting the behavior as mentally ill or psychotic. An action is incomprehensible to us if we cannot understand the motives, intentions, and thoughts of the person committing the behavior, or the customs or rules they are following in committing an action. Horwitz (1982) provided a number of examples from other cultures, one of which includes his description of how East African tribesman describe psychosis.

> *"There is one essential feature of African psychosis.*
> *Respondent after respondent qualifies his description of*
> *a psychotic behavior by saying "without reason." That is,*
> *murder as such is not psychotic. only murder without*
> *reason is psychotic."*

We have to only look at recent classifications of mass gun shooters as being "mad" or "deranged" to understand how relevant Horwitz's account of how we all label some as mentally ill based on incomprehensible behavior; it makes no sense to anyone. Sociologists attribute ideas about mental illness in the basic prerequisite of society and social interaction; we must be able to understand each other. While schizophrenia is found in all cultures, it may not be due to some hidden biological or neurological source, it may simply be that social interaction demands some sort of ability to take the role of the other, or to understand the perspective of the other person. When we cannot do this, the actions and behavior are incomprehensible, and the person is labeled as "insane" or "mad." Because the actions of the "madman" are incomprehensible, they are also unpredictable and consequently dangerous, all common attributes of the stereotypes we have of those with serious MHPs. Psychosis points to an altered sense of reality; the meaning of schizophrenia is not a split personality, but experiencing a second reality evidenced by delusions, hallucinations, and hearing voices. It is hard to talk to the person sitting next to you if you are not sharing the same conversation.

What is important to understand is that the comprehensibility of a behavior is culturally relevant, with each society or group defining what is normal and what is not. Behavior that an American might view as "odd" might be quite normal in another culture. Furthermore, it is important to take into account the social context within which behaviors occur. Historically, we have seen that those who hear voices and appear to communicate with the supernatural might be viewed as prophets or shamans, while today we would certainly label them as schizophrenic or psychotic. Social status and position are also important to labeling; those with less power are more likely to be labeled than those with more power.

Medicalization

An important sociological contribution to our understanding of mental health and distress is that of medicalization. Medicalization refers generally to the larger process of defining a nonmedical problem as a medical problem. In recent decades, mental health treatment has been driven by the medical model, more recently neuroscience, which combines the findings from several disciplines to understand the relationship between brain structure and human thoughts, feelings, and behaviors. Following diagnosis of the mental health disorder or disease, psychiatrists and therapists begin by prescribing a medication, which may help treat the symptoms but may not address the source of the MHP. Medicalization calls attention to the reality that the medical model can result in inappropriate medical treatment and a focus on individual pathology with little attention to the social factors that can create and shape the experience of illness. We can remind the readers of C. Wright Mills's comment in 1959 that many social problems are reduced to issues of individual pathology.

Medicalization was introduced by Peter Conrad in the 1970s when he wrote about the medicalization of hyperactivity in children (Conrad 2007). Hyperactivity involves a violation of acceptable norms about how children ought to behave and consequently was regarded as a form of deviance. In the 1980s, the American Psychiatric Association developed the diagnostic term attention deficit disorder (ADD), and children were diagnosed as either ADD or ADD with hyperactivity. A few years later, a new diagnostic label was developed, attention deficit hyper disorder or ADHD, and it was seen as a children's disorder that could persist into adulthood (see Box 1.1 for the common behaviors identified by the American Psychiatric Association for the diagnosis of ADHD).

BOX 1.1 Common Behaviors Associated with ADHD

Children exhibiting six symptoms of inattention and/or hyperactivity for six months, with behaviors occurring both at home and school, meet the diagnostic criteria for ADHD.

Inattention:

Often fails to pay close attention to details or makes careless mistakes.

Often has difficulty sustaining attention to tasks or play activities.

Often does not seem to listen when spoken to directly.

Often does not follow through on instructions and fails to finish chores.

Often has difficulty organizing tasks and activities.

Often avoids, dislikes, or is reluctant to engage in tasks that require sustained mental effort.

Is often easily distracted.

Is often forgetful.

Hyperactivity:

Often fidgets with hands, feet, or squirms.

Often stands or moves around when remaining seated as expected.

Often has difficulty playing quietly.

Often acts as if "driven by motor."

Often blurts out answers before questions have been completed.

Often interrupts or intrudes on others.

If we take a closer look at the behaviors originally associated with ADHD (and these have been expanded), it is easy to see how quickly the process of medicalization has taken over our understanding of "ordinary behavior" in children and adolescents. How many symptoms would you see in a typical child or teenager? Young people are impulsive and energetic by nature and have problems paying attention. The difficult role of parents and teachers is instilling the social norms for "appropriate behavior," which involves being quiet, not interrupting adults, sitting at a desk in school, and paying attention to the teacher for hours at a time. The diagnosis of ADHD has increased with more parents working, larger class sizes and fewer supports for teachers, less opportunities for "play" or sports, high-sugar diets, and increased emphasis on academic achievement. Research reported in the American Public Health Association June/July 2004 newsletter "The Nation's Health" summarized research published in *Pediatrics*, which showed a direct relationship between the number of hours children spent watching television and a diagnoses of ADHD. Furthermore, increased television before age three was associated with increased ADHD disorder by the age seven. The APHA summary cites co-author Frederick J. Zimmerman, who at that time was co-director of the Child Health Institute at the University of Washington, Seattle (www.apha.org/advocacy/releases/tvapril.pdf).

While originally limited to those under 18, the diagnosis of ADHD has been expanded to include adults, who largely self-diagnose before seeking treatment (Conrad 2007). The identification of ADHD and its expansion as a mental health disorder is itself evidence of medicalization. The reliance on medication to "treat" hyperactivity is further evidence of medicalization, as has been the continued increase in the numbers of children and adults diagnosed with ADHD. While only 40 years old, the diagnosis of ADHD is now one of the most prevalent psychiatric conditions. Originally, white boys in the United States were most likely to be diagnosed with ADHD, but the diagnoses now include a much wider range of young people as well as adults, providing further evidence of the role of medicalization. As yet we have not found a biological basis for ADHD, though many believe there is some genetic link. However, the behaviors typical of ADHD are not seen as social problems that influence normal childhood behaviors (high sugar diets, lack of exercise, long hours sitting in a desk or at the computer) or adult performance but as a medical problem with a medical fix in the form of medication. ADHD can also be viewed as a disability or dysfunction, but once again, it may be that the school system, the workplace, or the requirements of increased screen time with various devices and social media all work to produce inattention and hyperactivity. The major concern is that medical categories increasingly define what is normal and what is abnormal with expansion of medical categories and inclusion of many normal behaviors and responses as abnormal, leading to increased use of medications and medical treatment. In later chapters, we examine the role of the pharmaceutical industry in driving increased medicalization.

Concluding Thoughts

What is normal? Abnormal is defined as behavior that exists outside of a normal range. Emile Durkheim made the important sociological observation that "normal" is socially defined; it is what a given community views as appropriate behavior. We share the belief that meeting socially defined roles and rules that are defined by shared values and expectations is normative. Clearly, a key aspect of viewing mental health as "normal" results in an emphasis on conformity. While providing a broad-based framework for understanding mental health, the WHO (2022) definitions of mental health and illness maintain the long-standing dichotomy between healthy and sick, or normal versus abnormal, while refraining from the overt labels of sane versus insane. However, the WHO also emphasizes well-being and positive mental health, and avoids the overemphasis on a medical model of illness. Consequently, there is some pushback against the medicalization of what are widely viewed as social problems and increased understanding of the role of social context. However, stigma still persists and reduces support for needed social changes to our schools or workplaces to accommodate diversity in learning and work performance, especially for those with more serious MHPs.

Student Activities

1. The 2024 World Happiness Report was released in March of 2024 and widely discussed in the media. The report compares "happiness" in 150 countries, with the final average score going from 0 to 10 and weighted by a number of population factors. Of interest is how happiness is measured; it is not a

"ha ha" feeling good measure, but one of well-being. Finland has had the number one ranking in the past seven years, and in 2024, the United States had the lowest ranking. Globally, rates of well-being were the lowest for younger people. Explore the report and the data, focusing on differences between countries as well as age groups. Why are younger people "less happy"?

2. Explore images of people with mental illnesses, using the web, television, or print media. Provide examples of how those with an MHP are depicted in a stereotypical fashion. Do the examples exhibit incomprehensibility?

3. Recent data from the Centers of Disease Control in the United States find that one in nine children is now diagnosed with ADHD. Review data on ADHD reported by the Centers for Disease Control; examine differences in the diagnosis of ADHD by gender, race/ethnicity, or age. How prevalent is the diagnosis of ADHD among your peers?

References

Conrad, P. (2007). *The Medicalization of Society: On the Transformation of Human Conditions to Treatable Disorders.* Baltimore, Maryland: Johns Hopkins University Press.

Goffman, E. (1961). *Asylums: Essays on the Social Situation of Mental Patients and Other Inmates.* Garden City, NY: Doubleday Anchor Books.

Horwitz, A. (1982). *The Social Control of Mental Illness.* New York: Academic Press.

Mechanic, D. (2006). *The Truth About Health Care: Why Reform is Not Working in America.* New Brunswick, NJ: Rutgers University Press.

Mulvany, J. (2008). Disability, impairment or illness: The relevance of the social model of disability. *Sociology of Health and Illness.* 22 (5): 582–601.

Rosenhan, D. (1973). On being sane in insane places. *Science.* 179 (4070): 250–258.

Ryff, C. (1985). Happiness is everything, or is it? Explorations on the meaning of psychological well-being. *Journal of Personality and Social Psychology.* 57 (6): 1069–1081.

Scheff, T.J. (1984). *Being Mentally Ill: A Sociological Theory.* Chicago: Aldine.

Scull, A. (2023). Rosenhan revisited: Successful scientific fraud. *History of Psychiatry.* 34 (2): 180–195.

Slater, L. (2004). *Opening Skinners Box: Great Psychological Experiments of the Twentieth Century.* New York: WW Norton.

World Health Organization (WHO). (2022). *World Mental Health Report: Transforming Mental Health for All.*

CHAPTER 2

What Are the Sources of Mental Health Problems?

As we saw in Chapter 1, there is a good bit of disagreement over how we define and understand mental health problems (MHPs). A key issue continues to be what term we use to describe troublesome MHPs; are they illnesses, disorders, or conditions? Behind debates over how to define MHPs lays a more fundamental question: what is the cause of such MHPs? Whooley (2019, p. 22) argued that "mental distress has been, and remains, unknown" and that it may always be unknowable. This certainly applies not only to our understanding of schizophrenia but also to our approach to more common mental health conditions such as anxiety and depression when we cannot point to a single cause or "trigger." Given the shifting definitions of what mental distress is, there are contrasting theories about the causes of mental health conditions (referred to as its etiology) as well as in their treatment. The term "etiology" refers to theories about the causes of mental health conditions. In this chapter, we address diverse theories about the sources, or causes, of mental health conditions. In general, there have been three perspectives, or explanations, for mental health conditions: psychological or psychodynamic models, biomedical models, and sociological approaches. Both the psychological and biomedical approaches emphasize the individual as the source of the mental health conditions, while sociologists focus on the larger social context that shapes individual behavior.

To provide some clarity regarding definitions, in this text we will use the term mental health issues to refer to those with more acute mental health concerns; mental health conditions refer to more serious and disabling mental health issues; and MHPs refer to the more general category of both mental health issues and conditions. Therefore, we will most often use the term MHPs. Mental distress is a more widely used term we will use to refer to our everyday experience of distress as opposed to well-being.

Individualistic Explanations for MHPs

The etiology of mental illness or disorder is not yet understood or known, despite the widespread belief in a biological, genetic, or neurological model. Frances (2013, p. 23) argued there is neither a way to decide who is normal nor any useful definition of mental disorder. Even schizophrenia, a mental disorder that is widely assumed to have some genetic component, "is a construct, not a myth, not a disease. It is a description of a particular set of psychiatric problems, not an explanation of their cause." Psychological models were dominant until the 1970s and viewed mental health largely in terms of abnormal behavior, and courses in abnormal psychology are still prevalent and quite popular. There are diverse psychological approaches to abnormal behavior, all of which emphasize interpersonal interactions and family influences. The key to improved mental health lies in therapy, where the patient gains insight into how their life experiences have shaped their current behaviors. Psychoanalytical therapists focused on the role of the unconscious mind, following Freudian theory that emphasized the role of underlying unconscious drives and early life experiences. Abnormal behavior was seen as the result of getting "stuck" in one of the developmental stages or the defective use of various defensive mechanisms.

A much more widely utilized psychological approach is cognitive behavioral therapy, which focuses on how we think about our behaviors and emphasizes learning to think in new ways. Abnormal behavior occurs when our thoughts, or cognitive schemes, are not consistent or accurate or are based on a negative "lens." For example, a student may feel quite distressed with a C on an essay as a "poor" grade, or they could view this as the average grade, and hence more acceptable. Ideally, they will view the C as an opportunity to improve their performance to earn a better grade next time. The goal with cognitive behavior therapy is to change the way we not only think about a given situation, but also how we respond to it. A very common euphemism is to not focus on what is wrong with your life, but to emphasize what is positive (i.e. to view the glass as half-full rather than half-empty). Another powerful euphemism is when life throws you lemons, make lemonade. The goal of therapy is to teach more adaptive ways of thinking as well as concrete behaviors and strategies to cope with life's lemons.

While the role of psychotherapy has largely been replaced by a reliance on psychiatric medication, there is renewed emphasis on individual and family therapy with the crisis in youth mental health. Family therapy extends the one-on-one interaction between a therapist and individual to include relevant family members. Family therapy is important for children and adolescents and can be a critical addition to individual therapy when a young person is experiencing MHPs. Family-based therapy is especially important given that younger people (Gen Z) spend more time with family than previous cohorts. However, many therapists still look to biological sources and solutions for the MHP experienced by the child.

Since the 1980s, the biomedical model of mental disorders has been dominant, where mental health conditions are viewed as diseases or disorders. Mental health conditions are seen as having biological, biochemical, or neurological causes. Neuroscience combines the findings from several scientific disciplines to advance understanding of the relationship between brain structure and human behavior. Accordingly, increased reliance is placed upon neuroscience to diagnose mental disorders, and medication to provide treatment while psychotherapy is de-emphasized. Early researchers focused on genetics, and in the 1990s, funding for the Human Genome Project promised to find the genetic sources for a sizable number of both physical and mental health problems. However, we have not yet found a specific gene linked to MHPs and even research on schizophrenia points to the fundamental role of the environment in triggering a psychotic episode (Morgan, McKenzie and Fearon, 2008). The documentary *The Mysteries of Mental Illness* and Kolker's book *Hidden Valley Road* (see Appendix A) both do an excellent job of reviewing the evidence for biomedical and genetic explanations and concur in seeing that while progress has been made, we still lack a clear understanding of the etiology (or source) of MHPs.

Another approach has been in neurochemistry with a focus on neurotransmitters in the brain. Dopamine was thought to produce the symptoms of schizophrenia, and serotonin and norepinephrine played a role in depression. The evidence for the critical role of neurotransmitters came largely from pharmaceutical research, but these studies could not establish that faulty neurotransmission "caused" the symptoms or whether the symptoms caused the faulty wiring in the brain. In more statistical terms, just because two things are related (correlation) does not mean that one causes the other. It has been very difficult to establish biomedical causation for the majority of mental health conditions. A key problem is the realization of the complexity of how neurotransmitters interact. However, pharmaceutical advertising continues to advertise drugs that can "correct" the chemistry in our brains that is causing our MHPs. Students might explore more recent advertising on social media.

Another promising direction has been in neuroanatomy, which examines the structure of the brain. New technologies for brain imaging have allowed researchers to visualize how the brain functions. A cottage industry (a network of small companies often located in shopping malls) emerged in the early 2000s, which promised to pinpoint brain abnormalities at an early age. While subtle differences have been found in the brain structures, brain imaging has neither provided the kind of evidence needed for diagnosis or treatment, nor has it been useful in finding underlying sources that could prevent MHPs in the first place. Once again, while correlations exist, causation has not been established.

However, neurological advances in research have allowed us to understand how the social environment affects the brain. We now understand from research on the hippocampus region of the brain, which is the source of new cell growth, that the brain does respond to stress. With aging, new growth declines as one would expect. However, research has shown that stress also impairs new cell growth, leading to the kind of atrophy we see with old age. Further, stress also has an effect on those neurons in the brain, negatively affecting the connective wiring and feedback systems, resulting in brain damage. Stress also triggers depression, which then affects our hormonal system, leading to further complicated chemical effects on both the brain and the body. What we know is that emotions and the mind (neither of which have clear physical locations) do interact with both brain chemistry and structures, all of which are shaped by the social context that produces stress in the first place.

Sociological Approaches

Where does sociology fit in here? Sociologists agree with psychologists that mental health conditions need to be placed within an individual's experience of their social world, be that family, school, work, or historical trauma. While psychologists focus on the individual's adaption to their social context, sociologists focus on how the social context needs to be changed. Sociologists also have much to contribute to biomedical understanding of MHPs by contributing to the understanding of how biological factors (be they neurological or genetic) interact with the environment or social context. For example, while there may be a very well genetic component to depression, genes cannot explain cohort effects where both elderly and younger people experience higher rates of depression compared to those who are middle aged. What we refer to as the curvilinear relationship between age and depression is accounted for by differing environmental contexts, which is the social and historical sources of stress, as well as levels of mastery and social supports.

Sociologists can also add to our understanding of why we are so enamored with biological explanations for our distress, especially given the inconclusive evidence for biological cause of MHPs. Is the dominance of medical solutions due to our seeking a cure for every ill? The answer lies partly in our need to explain our own behaviors as well as not having much control over the social environments that lead to mental distress (for example we have no control over the weather or climate change). Sociologists also point to the role of insurance practices that require a specific diagnosis for reimbursement. Medication is often linked to determining a diagnosis in the place. If an antidepressant works, it must be depression; if an antipsychotic works, it must be psychosis; and if you are not sure, prescribe both, as we saw with Lauren Slater's experience in Chapter 1. Medication is cheaper than therapy and can be prescribed by primary health care providers. Another factor is the role of the pharmaceutical industry, which markets drugs to health care providers as well as patients via direct-to-consumer advertising.

Sociologists focus on the social context, with an emphasis on the larger macro or environmental sources of stress as well as understanding that social stress has different individual level impacts. COVID-19 provides a good example of both. COVID-19 was clearly a major source of what sociologists refer to as a structural strain, similar to that of a war or a major depression or recession. A structural strain has an impact on society at large with negative consequences for the economy, employment, health, and overall well-being. As a source of major structural strain, COVID-19 was beyond the control of any given individual and major changes were needed to compensate for the tremendous impact of COVID-19. We only need to reflect on the impact of COVID-19 on education and school as well as work with long-term consequences on our health still unknown. However, COVID-19 also had different individual impacts. Many of us, including medical staff, essential workers, and minorities, experienced significantly more COVID-19-related stress than other people did. We will see in Chapter 4 that stress is not equally distributed; those with less power and control over their work experienced higher levels of COVID-19-related stress, resulting in higher levels of mental distress. A good metaphor is from The Titanic, while we were all facing the same storm, we were not all in the same boat, and many did not even have access to a boat.

While stress research is inherently interdisciplinary (psychologists and biologists also study stress and there are research centers for the interdisciplinary study of stress), sociologists have a relatively novel approach to understanding MHPs, which is labeling or social reaction theory. Social reaction theory has traditionally viewed MHPs as deviance from widely accepted social norms, as described in Chapter 1. Social reactions to deviance involve labeling behavior as abnormal or normal. Labeling theory has been described as "radically sociological" because it views mental illness as "created and sustained by society itself" (Thoits, 2011, p. 121). The label of "mentally ill" involves negative stereotypes and is highly stigmatized, often resulting in outright discrimination. A stigma is an attribute that is discrediting and involves stereotypes. Countless surveys have demonstrated that many people believe those with mental illnesses are dangerous, unpredictable, can never be normal, cannot be talked with, and do not make good employees, which can result in social rejection and discrimination. Not only does the stigma of mental illness carry negative moral connotations, but also it can result in social isolation and withdrawal of the stigmatized individual from social interactions, leading to a host of negative consequences, including demoralization, unemployment, and homelessness.

Sociologists make an important distinction between public stigma and private or self-stigma. Public stigma involves stereotyping, prejudice, and discrimination – self-stigma is the internalization of public stigma and results in a devalued sense of self. Individuals who are labeled "mentally ill" internalize the negative attributes associated with the label and expect to be rejected, which is referred to as modified labeling theory. While a potentially positive effect of the label of mentally ill is the receipt of treatment or services, the self-stigma of the label has been found to lead to increased isolation and marginalization. This may be changing with wider social acceptance of MHPs, though it is likely that those with more stigmatized mental health conditions, such as schizophrenia, will continue to experience marginalization and rejection. We do know that today the public is more open to the recognition, treatment, and prevention of MHPs. However, the stigma associated with mental illness has not changed much over time. Sociologists have used the General Social Science Survey to compare public views of mental health conditions in the 1950s and 1996. The same question was repeated: "When you hear someone say a person is 'mentally ill' what does this mean to you?" The responses fit into four major categories: psychosis (breaks with reality), anxiety or depression, social deviance, or mental deficiency. Associating "mental illness" with psychosis and anxiety or depression had decreased, while associations with deviance and mental deficiency had increased. However, views of those with "mental illnesses" as dangerous including attributes of violence, frightening behavior (i.e. unstable, unpredictable, or uncontrollable) or violent psychosis has increased (Pescosolido, 2013). In short, in 1996, there was greater acceptance of "less serious" mental health conditions with greater fear of more serious mental health conditions. These trends have intensified, with an analysis of the 2018 General Social Science Survey finding less stigma associated with depression and anxiety, and greater stigma against those with schizophrenia with increased associations with dangerousness (Pescosolido et al., 2019. This is not surprising given widespread attention to acute MHPs (depression and anxiety) and the labeling of perpetrators of mass shooters as mentally ill.

An interesting question is whether the widespread belief that MHPs have a biological basis (i.e. they are a medical problem rather than one of deviant behaviors) has reduced the stigma of being labeled. While viewing mental illnesses as having a genetic basis has led to increased public support for treatment (especially medications), research has found that those who believe MHPs have a biological basis actually report higher level of stigma. Anderson and Harkness (2018) examined the multidimensional nature of stigmatized beliefs. They found that people hold diverse beliefs about mental illness, viewing mental illness as including chemical imbalance, genetic abnormality, bad character, or a consequence of stress. Stigma was assessed by "desired social distance" (i.e. how likely are you to want to avoid interactions with individuals with mental health conditions). Critically, the beliefs that were associated with stigma varied for different mental health conditions. Stress was more likely to be associated with depression and genetic factors with schizophrenia. A belief in a bad character did increase stigma, but only in accordance with other beliefs for a given condition. Pescosolido (2013, p. 15) concluded that "stigma is fundamentally a social phenomenon rooted in social relationships and shaped by the culture and structure of society."

Cultural Variability

The question of the universality or culturally specific nature of mental health conditions presents a test of the medical etiology, which asserts that the source of mental illness is biochemical, genetic, or neurological. If the cause is organic in nature, then such behaviors will be invariant across different cultures; that is mental health conditions would look the same in every culture with little gender, racial, or ethnic differences. If MHPs are in some part produced by social context, one would expect some degree of cultural variability in the prevalence and symptomology of behaviors and disorders characterized as mental illness or insanity. There would be variability both within and across countries and cultures. While some degree of MHPs is universal (i.e. all cultures characterize some forms of behavior as mental illness or disorder), there is a great deal of disagreement over whether specific categories of MHPs are indeed universal.

Only schizophrenia has some evidence of universality, with every society having an incidence rate of around 1% of the population experiencing symptoms of psychosis, hallucinations, and delusions.

However, the array of symptoms displayed by individuals diagnosed with schizophrenia is remarkably diverse and complex with no two people having the same set of symptoms. Consequently, the diagnosis of schizophrenia is culturally variable. An early comparison of the United States and the United Kingdom found that in the face of similar symptoms of psychoses, psychiatrists in the United States were more likely to diagnose schizophrenia and those in the United Kingdom were more likely to diagnose manic depression (Cooper, 1972). While cross-cultural research challenges the widely held belief that schizophrenia is a biomedical disease, it does demonstrate that the social environment influences both the course and the outcome of psychosis (Morgan, McKenzie, and Fearon, 2008). That is, the social and cultural context influences both symptoms and the response to symptoms of psychosis.

Not surprising, there is a great deal of cultural variability in more "common" or normal mental health issues. Kleinman and Goode's classic (1985) cross-cultural study of depression found that symptoms of depression vary, as does the experience of sadness, failure, and loss. In fact, many societies or cultures did not even have words or labels to describe depression. In Japan, "utsubyo" (depression) was seen as a rare disorder, which prevented people from living a normal life (Watters, 2010). The American view of depression is related to a more individualized focus on emotion and self, while in Japan, the individual is seen as dependent on others and society. Feeling sad is unavoidable and also viewed as a mark of strength. However, economic pressures in the 1990s led to an increase in suicides in Japan and people began to see stress as a source of depression, not just sadness or grief. Drug companies took advantage of this change in cultural beliefs and created a market for antidepressants to cope with depression, labeling depression as "the cold of the soul" (Watters, 2010).

Social conditions and environments are critical in not only understanding what constitutes a MHP, but also in the course and outcome of MHPs. Early research in the 1930s found that rates of schizophrenia increased in cities, and more recent research has found that not only living in a city, but also the years living in a city were associated with higher diagnoses of schizophrenia. In addition, research has documented that individuals with a diagnosis of schizophrenia do better in less developed countries. While the mechanisms by which the social environment influences mental health have not been thoroughly studied, it is likely that the higher levels of stress and lower social supports in industrialized societies are critical (Morgan, Mckenzie, and Fearon, 2008). An important distinction in understanding cross-cultural differences in mental health is the degree of social cohesion. Individualist societies value autonomy and individual rights, but generate higher levels of isolation and loneliness, and individuals with MHPs experience more symptom severity and poorer rates of relapse and recovery. Communal societies provide greater group cohesion and social supports; consequently, individuals with even severe mental conditions such as schizophrenia do better over time.

At the same time, globalization is reducing cultural variability. Watters (2010) provided a number of examples of the ways in which conceptions of mental health and treatment have been "westernized." In China, girls began to model their appearance norms to fit western standards for beauty, leading to anorexia. Research on schizophrenia in Zanzibar shows how there had been widespread acceptance of those who experienced psychosis. However, "westernization" resulted in an increased reliance on a medicalized approach to treatment. Levels of stigma increased and those with schizophrenia began to be viewed as dangerous and were subsequently excluded from family and their social networks. The analysis of PTSD in Sri Lanka after the 2004 tsunami demonstrates that collectivist and individualist societies have very different understandings of stress and how to deal with stress. More individualistic countries have much to learn from more communal or collectivist societies, especially in the wake of COVID-19. Did COVID-19 bring us together or did it isolate us? Time will tell and comparative research is needed to see the impact of COVID-19 on diverse societies.

Concluding Thoughts

As this overview should indicate, there is much more research that needs to be done to extend our understanding of mental health and illness before we will be able to resolve the ongoing debates over the existence and causes of mental illnesses, much less on suitable treatments. We do know that social conditions and environments are critical in not only understanding what constitutes a MHP, but in the course and outcome of MHPs as well. However, the mechanisms through which the social environment influences mental health have not been thoroughly studied. Moreover, COVID-19 certainly changed our ideas about what is normal by upending what had been "normal" prior to COVID as MHPs reached epidemic proportions worldwide. Neither biology, psychology, nor sociology can provide a complete understanding of mental health and mental health conditions. Instead, a biopsychosocial model is necessary, which realizes there are complex interactions between underlying biological conditions, psychological processes, and social influences. A biopsychosocial approach is clearly in accord with recent research that examines how growth promoters in the brain, which are the biological sources of resiliency, are influenced by not only genetics but also early childhood trauma, current levels of stress, and the lifelong accumulation of stress. The research on how the brain reacts to stress actually fits well with the research on neurotransmitters. This finding is not really so novel, as we have known for some time that stress weakens the immune system. While there is certainly a biochemical mechanism at work here, we may never have a concise explanation for mental health conditions given the complexity of the interaction between our bodies, how we think, and how we respond to environmental stressors. Furthermore, understanding the interaction between physical and mental processes is muddled, and recent research on complex trauma and the long-term impacts of COVID-19 provides more questions than answers. In a recent book, *The Weight of the Future: How a Changing Climate Changes Our Brains*, Clayton Page Aldern (a Rhodes Scholar and neuroscientist turned journalist) argues that climate change has had an effect on our minds, moods, and brains. Certainly, many of us experience climate anxiety, which can be seen as a normal response to a real threat. While we may not be able to control for the sources of stress, we can indeed improve how we deal with stress.

Student Activities

1. Look back over the COVID-19 years and your own experience of MHPs (which can include those of members of your family or friends). What factors contributed to poorer mental health? What role do you think psychological, biological, or sociological factors played? How did they interact (i.e. do you see the strength in the biopsychosocial approach)?

2. Examine advertising for common mental health conditions (and maybe compare television, print in magazines, and online). What views of the etiology of MHPs are prevalent?

3. Look at your own community and provide an assessment of whether it is more individualistic or communal, and more urban or rural. How is life different in a city compared to a more rural area? What are the implications of where you live for understanding mental health and distress?

References

Anderson, M. and Harkness, S.K. (2018). When do biological attributions of mental illness reduce stigma? *Society and Mental Health*. 8 (3): 175–194.

Cooper, B. (1972). Sociology in the context of social psychiatry. *British Journal of Psychiatry*. 161 (5): 594–598.

Frances, A. (2013). *Saving Normal: An Insider's Revolt Against Out-of-Control Psychiatric Diagnosis, DSM-5, Big Pharma, and the Medicalization of Ordinary Life*. New York: Harper Collins.

Kleinman, A. and Good, B. (1985). *Culture and Depression: Studies in the Anthropology and Cross-Cultural Psychiatry of Affect and Disorder*. Berkely, CA: University of California Press.

Morgan, C., McKenzie, K. and Fearon, P. (2008). *Society and Psychosis*. Cambridge: Cambridge University Press.

Pescosolido, B.A. (2013). The public stigma of mental illness: What do we think; what do we know; what can we prove? *Journal of Health and Social Behavior*. 54 (1): 1–21.

Pescosolido, B.A., Manago, B. and Monahan, J. (2019). Trends in public stigma of mental illness in the US, 1996–2018. *JAMA Network Open*. 4 (12): e2140202.

Thoits, P.A. (2011). Mechanisms linking social ties and support to physical and mental health. *Journal of Health and Social Behavior*. 52 (2): 145–161.

Watters, E. (2010). *Crazy Like Us: The Globalization of the American Psyche*. New York, NY: The Free Press.

Whooley, O. (2019). *On The Heels of Ignorance: Psychiatry and the Politics of Not Knowing*. Chicago, Illinois: University of Chicago Press.

CHAPTER 3

Assessing Mental Health and Distress

In order to arrive at estimates of how many people suffer from mental health conditions, there needs to be some way to determine who has a mental health condition and who does not. This is not as simple as one might expect and there are two different approaches to the assessment of mental health and distress. First, there are theories that conceptualize health and illness as opposites, a categorical dichotomy, where a person is labeled as either sick or well based on clearly defined diagnostic criteria. When experiencing a mental health problem (MHP), we want to know if we have a diagnosis of depression, anxiety, or some other condition. Second, there are theories that view mental health and illness in terms of a continuum, with health and illness at opposite ends of the poles, and most of us falling somewhere in between. In other words, there are varying degrees of wellness and distress. With a diagnosis you are either sick or not, with a continuum you will fall somewhere between a low number to a higher number with a greater degree of variability.

Beyond assessing which individuals are mentally well or not, we also need to determine how many people experience mental health conditions, a process commonly referred to as population estimates. Epidemiology refers to the study of the distribution of illness in a population, and social epidemiologists examine existing data as well as conducting population-based surveys. Epidemiological research not only assesses overall rates of illness, but also identifies which groups have higher rates of particular conditions, which can lead to an understanding of the specific causes of a disorder or disease. Epidemiologists have advanced degrees in the social sciences, and

BOX 3.1 Epidemiological Terms

Morbidity is the prevalence of diseases in a population, whereas comorbidity is the co-occurrence of illness or conditions and associated risk factors.

Point prevalence refers to the percentage of the population affected with an illness or condition at a given point of time.

Lifetime prevalence refers to the percentage of the population *ever* affected with an illness or condition.

Incidence rate is the rate at which new cases of an illness or disorder form in the population; for example, many are now concerned with the prevalence rate at which depression is found among all age groups and the fact that incidence rates seem to be increasing for young women.

sociologists have played a leading role in collecting both individual and population level data. In assessing mental disorders, there are a variety of terms the student needs to be familiar with (see Box 3.1)

Diagnostic Classification

Medical science and psychiatry are organized around elaborate, formal systems of diagnoses or an array of dichotomous indicators of whether or not a person has one or more particular illnesses or disorders. The World Health Organization (WHO) uses the International Classification of Disease, currently the 2019 version 11 (ICD-11). The WHO generally uses the term "mental health condition," but when describing the epidemiology and prevalence of mental health, they use the term "mental health disorder," as the ICD is based upon the assessment of a diagnostic disorder that meets clinical standards. International data are collected with the WHO's Global Health Estimates and the 2019 Global Burden of Disease, Injuries and Risk Factors Study conducted by the Institute of Health Metrics and Evaluation. These data provide estimates of the prevalence of mental disorder across countries, as well as information about differences by age and sex. The data are limited to the quality of information provided by each country, which can be incomplete for various reasons. Collecting epidemiological data requires an investment in public health, which is beyond the means of many poorer countries.

In the United States, the major sources of information on the epidemiology of mental health are the Centers for Disease Control and Prevention (CDC) and the Substance Abuse and Mental Health Services Administration (SAMHSA), which also use categorical measures of mental disorder. The standard for the diagnoses of mental disorders is the American Psychiatric Association's (APA) *Diagnostic and Statistical Manual* (DSM). The DSM is used in clinical practice as well as in a great deal of epidemiological research to determine whether or not someone has a mental disorder and to provide population level data about the prevalence of mental disorders. Currently, in version 5, the *DSM* provides the classification system by which clinicians and researchers can identify and diagnose distinct mental disorders. These disorders are assumed to be discrete, that is, they do not overlap with one another. The classification of mental disorders is referred to as psychiatric nosology and has generated a great deal of controversy (Frances, 2013).

Sociologists have demonstrated that the *DSM* overstates the amount of mental disorder, viewing all evidence of psychiatric symptoms, regardless of their cause, as evidence of pathology. An extended illustration of this process is provided in Horwitz and Wakefield's 2007 book (*The Loss of Sadness*), which is critical of the classification of "normal sadness" as a DSM depressive disorder. The problem is that the DSM does not take into account contextual factors (the social context), which may account for the existence of various symptoms of so-called depression. A more recent book by Horwitz and Wakefield (2012) examines anxiety. Rates of anxiety have been increasing with close to half of the US adult population suffering from anxiety at some point in their lives, which is the lifetime prevalence rate. This does not mean that half of us are right now experiencing anxiety, which would be the point prevalence. Of interest in the incidence rate, how many new cases of anxiety are there? No doubt the incidence rate increased during COVID-19, leading to higher lifetime prevalence rates. The question is which groups have experienced the greatest increases in anxiety, something we will return to later in the chapter.

Revisions to the most recent version of the DSM were especially contentious, and the roots of this controversy and the ensuing political battles over DSM-5 are described by Francis (2013). A key critique has been that with each revision of the DSM, more and more conditions are defined as "abnormal," a process Frances describes as diagnostic inflation. Diagnostic inflation is driven in part by

BOX 3.2 Diagnostic Inflation in the Diagnostic and Statistical Manual (DSM)

Volume	Year	No. of Diagnoses	No. of Pages
Vol 1	1952	106	130
Vol II	1968	182	134
Vol III	1980	265	494
Vol IIIR	1987	292	567
Vol IV	1994	297	886
DSM-5	2013	298	992

medicalization and in part by the pharmaceutical industry, which profits from the use of medication to treat ordinary, or normal, conditions. Medicalization occurs when nonmedical problems (such as sadness) come to be defined in medical terms (such as major depressive disorder), and there is increased reliance on psychiatric medications for more and more "conditions" (such as anxiety). In Box 3.2, we summarize data reported in Suris, Holiday and North (2016) who provide a concise review of the history and changes in the classification of disorders.

In response to criticisms of DSM-5, the National Institute of Mental Health proposed a new classification system to be used by researchers as opposed to clinicians, who will continue to use DSM-5 in their diagnosis of patients. The Research Domain Criteria (RDoC) system is based upon the assumption that mental distress is primarily a problem residing in the brain, and research should focus on genetics and neuroscience. Consequently, the RDoC represents an increased medicalization as well as further decontextualization of mental disorder and distress (Whooley, 2014).

Of interest is how different groups utilize the DSM, a question addressed in Schnittker's 2017 book. Schnittker contrasts how researchers, clinicians, and the public actually use the DSM. Researchers rely on the DSM to arrive at population estimates of the incidence and prevalence of mental health disorders. In contrast, clinicians are focused on the patient and the experience of MHPs, which they generally believe are core features of our individual psyche, though not well understood. Clinicians are more interested in treatment than diagnosis, and treatment often helps identify a given disorder. Hence, clinicians diagnose fewer disorders than researchers do. Clinicians are also subject to pressures related to reimbursement; insurance companies generally require a diagnosis in order to authorize treatment. The example Schnittker provides is attention deficit hyperactivity disorder (ADHD), which is widely overdiagnosed. Why? Because the criteria are so vague that most young people exhibit some symptoms of ADHD such as restlessness and inability to concentrate (see a list of symptoms in Chapter 1). At the same time parents want improved academic performance; teachers prefer "well-behaved" students and the medications prescribed meet all these criteria and are quickly approved by insurance plans. Consequently, the DSM is "caught in the middle of these economic and policy trends" (p. 133). Another example is post-traumatic stress disorder (PTSD). In both cases, clinicians are pressured to make a diagnosis but tend to overlook other diagnoses or symptoms that do not fit the primary diagnosis, which is widely accepted. The bottom line is that while clinicians are focused on treatment, for insurance purposes, they have to supply a diagnosis.

What about the public? Schnittker finds that the public focuses on context; they want to know what factors lead to an MHP. Is an individual suffering from grief (normal sadness) or clinical depression without an adequate contextual explanation? For the public, help seeking is critical; most of us do not seek out professional help until we have decided we do have an MHP, which involves labeling: self-labeling as well as labeling by others. Schnittker reviews the evidence available about changes in public beliefs, comparing responses to vignettes in the General Social Survey from 1996 to 2006. A quick takeaway is that the general public increasingly adheres to a medical view of MHPs, as evidenced by the following trends Schnitker identified.

1. The public in 2006 was more likely to identify symptoms described in the vignettes as a mental illness and not a result of the "ups and downs of normal life."
2. These symptoms were more likely to be seen as evidence of a disease (i.e. acceptance of biomedical explanations for the problem).

3. Yet, the public also accepts environmental explanations and recognizes the role of stress in producing MHPs.

4. In terms of treatment, if the MHP is viewed as biomedical, then the public supports specialty mental health treatment. If environmental (i.e. stress), then less focus is placed on the need for treatment.

For example, take a woman whose husband dies unexpectedly at the age of 62 years in his first year of retirement. While her physician recommended an antidepressant, she declines it. She is willing to take a sleeping pill for a week or so to help her sleep, but did not feel she needed counseling or therapy. Instead, she joined a group of divorced and widowed women and reached out to her family and friends for support. Another woman may find herself unable to stop crying and retreats from contact with her friends and family. An antidepressant may help this woman cope with her grief.

While death is "normal" even when unexpected, our experience of grief is variable and can lead to anxiety and depression as well as physical symptoms such as nausea, headaches, and increased blood pressure, all of which can weaken the immune system. Of interest is determining whether a given response to grief is normal or not, with a new DSM diagnosis finding that long-term grief may itself constitute a mental disorder. Referred to as prolonged grief disorder, the criteria are intense pain a year after the loss and an inability to resume past activities. Naming prolonged grief as pathological does not acknowledge the reality that grief and loss is complex, and the pain of losing a grandparent cannot compare to the pain of a child's suicide. The American Psychological Association provides guidelines for coping with grief, which are in accordance with more general clinical guidelines for dealing with mental distress: adequate diet and hydration, sleep, exercise, and seeking social supports. Grief is not something to get over, or to be cured, but involves a process of healing that cannot always be reduced to a year.

Continuous Measures of Mental Health and Distress

An alternative to the DSM are continuous assessments of mental health and mental distress, such as scales to assess psychological well-being. Scales and indices assess not only the problem but also the severity and frequency along a continuum. The psychosocial model of mental illness (dominant until the 1970s) was based upon a continuum definition of mental health and illness where the boundary between health and illness was fluid and subject to social and environmental influences. That is, it was widely accepted that anyone could become "sick" if subject to the right conditions or environmental stressors. An advantage of continuous measures is that we can assess not only negative outcomes but also positive ones, which are clearly important to overall mental health and well-being.

Many sociologists use various continuous measures in their research on mental health. A measure of mental distress that is commonly used is the Kessler 6 index (K6). The K6 assesses the frequency with which people experience sadness, nervousness, restlessness, worthlessness, hopelessness, and feeling that everything is an effort. The National Health Interview Survey (NHIS) has been assessing mental health since 1997 and provides for an assessment of mental health trends. The NHIS is a nationally representative household interview survey of adults and children, which is collected throughout the year by Census interviewers. Adults are asked whether they regularly had feelings of worry, nervousness, or anxiety as well as feelings of depression with responses being between "a little" and "a lot" or somewhere in between. In 2019, 11% of respondents felt anxious and 4.7% reported feelings of depression. In 2022, rates of anxiety had increased somewhat to 12.5% and depression to 4.95%. Amy Johnson (2021) analyzed changes in psychological distress for adults over 20 years (1997–2017). She found that psychological distress had not changed much over those 20 years, with scores in the middle of the range from low to high. However, she did find age differences, with younger adults having the highest levels of distress, with lower distress after age 50, but increasing after age 70.

It is also important to assess positive mental health or well-being, which includes purpose, fulfillment, mastery, and self-esteem. These kinds of measures help us understand the reality of people's lives and how social context can shape mental health and distress. Keyes (2017) has developed a continuum model of mental health, which ranges from languishing to flourishing. The "Complete State Model" follows the WHO in viewing mental health as the absence of disease and including indicators of positive mental health and well-being. However, in addition to assessing emotional well-being and psychological well-being, Keyes (see Box 3.3) developed indicators of social well-being, which include social acceptance, social coherence, social contribution, social growth, and social integration.

BOX 3.3 The Mental Health Continuum Short Form

During the past month, how often did you feel:

(Never, once or twice, almost once a week, 2–3 times a week, almost every day, every day)

Emotional well-being:

1. Happy
2. Interested in life
3. Satisfied with life

Social well-being:

Social contribution: that you had something important to contribute to society

Social integration: that you belonged to a community (social group, school, and neighborhood)

Social growth: that our society is a good place, or is becoming a better place, for all people

Social acceptance: that people are basically good

Social coherence: that the way society works made sense to you

Psychological well-being:

Self-acceptance: that you liked most parts of your personality

Environmental mastery: that you are good at managing the responsibilities of your daily life

Positive relations with others: that you had warm and trusting relationships with others

Personal growth: that you had experiences that challenged you to grow and become better

Autonomy: that you are confident to think or express your own ideas and opinions

Purpose in life: that your life has a sense of direction or meaning

Source: Adapted from Keyes (2017).

Keyes' model moves sociologists well beyond debates over the validity of diagnostic criteria to a more useful approach to understanding the mental health profile of a given community or population. In research using the long form of the Mental Health Continuum as well as a diagnostic tool to assess major depression, panic attacks, and generalized anxiety, Keyes (2017) examined changes in mental health between 1995 and 2005. While overall prevalence rates of both mental health and distress were relatively stable, there were changes in individual experiences of languishing and flourishing over time. Only half of the adults who were flourishing in 1995 were flourishing in 2005, while only 45% of those who were languishing in 1995 were languishing in 2005. This research demonstrates that our mental health "state" is dynamic and changes over time. What we need to pay attention to are increases in overall prevalence rates of mental distress (as we have seen with COVID-19) and ways to promote positive mental health and well-being. Inclusion of social indicators of social well-being is clearly important to understanding where promotion efforts should be targeted. For example, the 2022 WHO report emphasizes social and emotional learning in schools to promote better mental health among young people.

An alternative approach is offered by Schnittker (2017), the network approach, which is based on the connections between symptoms. Rather than focusing on the causes of mental disorders, the network approach sees the relations between symptoms as being linked with each other, rather than reflecting some underlying cause. With a network approach we can examine the pathways between symptoms, how some symptoms can lead to other symptoms, and how symptoms may overlap with one another. For example, different groups may respond to similar stressors with very different symptoms. We know that men are more likely to externalize distress, with higher rates of substance use; women are more likely to internalize stress, with higher rates of depression.

With a network approach, the wide individual variability seen in MHPs such as depression (eating too much or too little, sleeping too much or too little, feeling sad, angry, or numb) can be better understood and explained. Further, a network approach does a much better job of explaining why symptoms of anxiety are found in a majority of the DSM diagnoses. Some symptoms may serve as connecting bridges, and by using a network approach, we can identify the core features of mental distress and how they can lead to more disabling mental disorders.

The network approach described by Schnittker fits with ideas about mental health conditions being aligned on a spectrum. A spectrum refers to a wide range of variation and is not the same as a scale or index that examines similar symptoms (i.e. how often do you feel nervous). Originating in ideas about autism spectrum disorder and fitting newer ideas about neurodiversity, differences in "symptoms" or "functioning" do not reflect an underlying mental disorder or pathological condition. In terms of autism spectrum disorder, the focus is on the degree of disability with a ranking of Level 1 (needs some support), Level 2 (needs substantial support), and Level 3 (needs very substantial support). The need for supports will vary over time and are influenced by the social context, for example, family and school. Children in the United States with autism spectrum disorder have been eligible for additional educational supports based on their degree of disability.

Neurodiversity is an alternative to the medical model of disability that has dominated child psychiatry and its approach to autism spectrum disorder. As described by Elizabeth Pellirano and Jacqueline den Houting in their 2021 paper in *The Journal of Child Psychology and Psychiatry*, the medical paradigm is based on ideas about deficiency. Autism has been described as a series of persistent deficits, with a focus on individual behaviors, which often results in autistic people being seen as less than human. Neurodiversity was first coined by autistic sociologist Judy Singer and the journalist Harvey Blume in 1998 to refer to the range of diversity that exists in neurological development. Most of us are neurodiverse with a range of typical and divergent ways of thinking and behaving (Pellirano and den Houting, 2021, p. 386). The important point is that diversity is valuable in its own right and what have been labeled as "deficits" are often strengths or even innovative ways to deal with new situations.

Transgender advocates have also rejected the DSM diagnosis of Gender Identity Disorder, emphasizing that variance in gender identity is normal. While the DSM-5 now uses the term gender dysphoria, there remain concerns over whether trans people will be able to access mental and physical healthcare. Recognizing the wide range of human neurodiversity may reduce pathologizing behaviors seen as "abnormal" and will also reduce stigma. This is where a social model of disability, which emphasizes the need for society to change to meet human diversity, is a better framework for promoting mental health. For children and young adults coping with autism or gender identity, mainstream school settings may be an inaccessible context for learning (Pellirano and den Houting, 2021, p. 387). Such settings may not promote individual flourishing, much less the wider social goals of inclusion and equity. Neurodiversity is an important and emerging social justice movement and can certainly empower young people to change the systems that exclude them.

The Crisis in Anxiety

Rates of anxiety have been rising for the last 20 years (Horwitz and Wakefield, 2012), although the NHIS data show that the increases are incremental. However, anxiety has increased with COVID-19, especially among younger people. A sociological approach to anxiety is offered by Schnittker (2021) who demonstrates the ways in which anxiety is shaped by the social environment and social factors. Social context is critical, so we will focus on anxiety among college students and young people. While college students have had increased rates of anxiety since the 1950s, these rates have accelerated in recent years, with over half of college students reporting feeling overwhelming anxiety, according to survey data from the American College Health Association and the Healthy Minds Study. Students face numerous concerns over their performance, including math anxiety, exam anxiety, and writing anxiety. Sheila Tobias introduced the idea of math anxiety in 1976 in Ms. Magazine and published a book in 1978, *Overcoming Math Anxiety*. Math anxiety was gendered, with woman (at that time, often new to college) more likely to experience it.

Today, we have more minority and first-generation college students facing new pressures to perform. The smartphone generation may not be as well prepared and Twenge (2017) documents the role that social media has played in greater social isolation, less connectedness, less sleep, and less time doing homework and reading. Another social psychologist, Jonathan Haidt in his book *The Anxious Generation: How the Great Rewiring of Childhood in Causing an Epidemic of Mental Illness* (Penguin Books), argues that the increases in anxiety coincide with the rise of a phone-based childhood, targeting the period between 2010 and 2015 as one of rapid social changes (review of the book and interview with the author in the *New York Times Book Review* April 21, 2024). Changes in how young people relate to each other via cell phones and social media may also generate greater uncertainty and anxiety (Schnittker, 2021).

There are also many wider social forces that can cause anxiety, including climate change, social and civil unrest, calls for social justice, and political polarization. There has been a focus on what psychologists refer to as eco-anxiety or the fear of environmental doom brought on by climate change. We have witnessed increased worldwide devastation due to hurricanes, floods, and wildfires. Many colleges are dealing with student protests over the situation in Gaza, with conflicts between Palestine and Israeli groups. College students are confronting the reality of how the world works, and does not, in their classes and on campus. Feeling unsettled, nervous, jittery, or fearful of the uncertain future is a "normal" response, as is anger. It can also lead to efforts to redress the source of anxiety; for example, becoming active in climate activism or racial justice, or simply volunteering at the local homeless shelter. However, intense and never-ending anxiety is certainly a risk factor for both depression and suicide. Let's look more closely at anxiety, drawing from Horwitz and Wakefield's 2012 book, *All We Have to Fear is Fear*.

Anxiety was introduced by Freud as neurasthenia, a nervous condition applied to women, and more widely referred to as hysteria. Freud's criteria for anxiety as an inappropriate response to danger were incorporated into the first DSM, which "used anxiety as the central conceptual principle behind all psychoneurotic disorders" (Horwitz and Wakefield, 2012, p. 93). However, DSM-III and DSM-IIIR transformed the diagnoses of anxiety and replaced the contextual requirement (i.e. perception of a given threat) to the more general criteria of feeling anxious. Anxiety is an emotion, but it is a forward-looking emotion where we anticipate the future (how am I going to pass this class). Depression can be seen as a response to past events (I failed the core class in biology and do not know what to do). We can see here how looking at the connections between symptoms over time (the network approach) may provide more insights into MHPs than a simple diagnosis would provide.

There are eight categories of anxiety: specific phobia, social phobia (also referred to as social anxiety disorder), agoraphobia, panic disorder, PTSD, acute stress disorder, obsessive–compulsive disorder, and generalized anxiety disorder. Generalized anxiety disorder is excessive anxiety and worry occurring more days than not for six or more months. Here we see how DSM diagnoses involve both the duration and frequency of symptoms, but also does not include the context within which the anxiety occurs. We can anticipate that first-generation college students will experience anxiety as the first semester finals loom ahead, but those questions are not addressed with the DSM. Likewise, social phobia was also decontextualized in revisions to the DSM, with increasing rates as a result. The diagnosis of obsessive–compulsive disorder as a type of anxiety was, and still is, debated. PTSD is controversial as it is the only DSM disorder that acknowledges the role of social context. However, the DSM criteria are so general (experiencing a traumatic event, including witnessing someone being injured or killed, which is likely in combat, a natural disaster, a life-threatening accident, or the sudden unexpected death of a loved one) that almost all of us will meet the criteria for PTSD at some time in our lives. Do we need medication? Not always, and responses to common traumas can result in resiliency and post-traumatic growth. However, the DSM does not provide for classification of positive mental health.

While "normal" levels of anxiety may be high, there is a wide degree of cultural variability in how we express and respond to anxiety. Grinker (2021, p. 169) argues that PTSD suits more individualist cultures, a finding collaborated by Waters' (2010) account of how PTSD was not applicable to the experience of Sri Lankains following the tsunami of 2004. Instead of counseling and therapy, stress was resolved by collective group activities and greater social bonding. There are also evolutionary influences, and many phobias have been linked to concrete environmental threats (heights, darkness, snakes). Social anxiety may be a response to the relatively new urban environment with large crowds and new places. As our social environment changes, so will the roots of our anxiety, as we see with college students. Seeking help is okay if the anxiety overwhelms us. As Horwitz and Wakefield argue (2012, p. 223), "there is nothing wrong with using therapy to help people adjust to social demands... However, misrepresenting normal fears as mental disorder is incorrect." However, in order to get reimbursement for therapy, you will probably need a DSM diagnosis.

There are additional instruments used to assess anxiety in young people. The Multidimensional Anxiety Scale for Children (MASC), now in its second edition, is widely used by counselors in schools to screen those between the age of 8 and 19 years for a broad range of symptoms of anxiety. The MASC2 can also be used by parents or young people who can download the manual for a small fee. The original MASC contained 39 items, and the second edition has 50 items that ask about a wide range of physical and emotional symptoms. Horwitz and Wakefield (2012) find that many of the symptoms of anxiety are fairly normal feelings for adolescents, such as nervousness, tenseness, embarrassment, and stomach aches. As with the DSM, the MASC2 has been found to be reliable, but it also does not provide for the identification of the contexts of the symptoms that are reported. While certainly useful for early identification of potentially serious mental health conditions (in which case the screening should be followed by a clinical interview), there is potential to view normal intense teenage angst as pathological. School and community-based emotional learning programs can certainly be used to teach young people how to cope with anxiety as well as the sources of stress, which create anxiety.

Concluding Thoughts

The fact that there is no consensus on the definition of what we mean by mental "illness" or on the sources, causes or etiology, of MHPs should not be surprising that there are diverse ways to assess mental health conditions. However, it is important to have reliable data as to how many people actually experience MHPs so we can provide adequate treatment and supports. In this chapter, we introduced readers to the distinction between dichotomous and continuous measures. We also described some new approaches that examine variability in terms of a spectrum or neurodiversity as well as the network approach that examines connections between symptoms. The WHO uses the ICD-11, which is based on the DSM classification of mental disorders. In the United States, the CDC and the NHIS provide yearly estimates of population levels of mental health, and we can see that over time, rates of mental distress are relatively stable, but with increases in anxiety, especially among younger people. Accordingly, we provided more information on the assessment of anxiety. Sociologists utilize more continuum measures of mental distress and have also prioritized assessment of the social sources of mental well-being. Sociologists also argue that the experience of mental health and distress are linked to our social context and emphasize that medical models of mental illness decontextualize the sources of these conditions. In the following chapter, we describe the dominant framework in sociology for understanding mental health – the Stress Process Model.

Student Activities

1. Examine recent data on Mental Health from the Centers for Disease Control and Prevention and the WHO. How does the United States compare to the rest of the world in terms of prevalence and mental health and distress? Select your own country and provide information on the conditions that are shaping mental health.

2. Examine recent reports and data on Youth Mental Health (globally, regionally, or locally). Provide a comparison of national and global data and also look for data closer to your own "home," be that a state or province, or a rural or urban environment. Provide a summary and discuss the larger social context that has shaped the youth mental health crisis in your own community.

3. Working in groups, administer Keyes' Mental Health Continuum Short Form (Box 3.3) to a defined groups of college students on your campus or in your community. What did you expect to find? What did you find? What impacts do you think social media has on the components of well-being identified by Keyes?

References

Frances, A. (2013). *Saving Normal: An Insiders Revolt against Out-of-Control Psychiatric Diagnosis, DSM-5, Big Pharma, and the Medicalization of Ordinary Life*. New York, NY: HarperCollins.

Grinker, R.R. (2021). *Nobody's Normal: How Culture Created the Stigma of Mental Illness*. New York, NY: WW Norton & Company.

Horwitz, A.V. and Wakefield, J.C. (2012). *All We Have to Fear is Fear: Psychiatry's Transformation of Natural Anxieties into Mental Disorders*. New York, NY: Oxford University Press.

Johnson, A. (2021). Changes in mental health treatment, 1997–2017. *Journal of Health and Social Behavior*. 62 (1): 53–68.

Keyes, C. (2017). The dual continuum model: The foundation for a sociology of mental health and illness. In: *The Handbook for the Study of Mental Health*, 3e (ed. T.L. Scheid and E.R. Wright), pp. 66–82. Cambridge, UK: Cambridge University Press.

Pellirano, E. and den Houting, J. (2021). Annual research review: Shifting from "normal science" to neurodiversity in autism science. *The Journal of Child Psychology and Psychiatry.* 63 (4): 381–396. doi: org/10.111/jcpp. 13534

Schnittker, J. (2017). *The Diagnostic System Why the Classification of Psychiatric Disorders is Necessary, Difficult, and Never Settled.* New York, NY: Columbia University Press.

Schnittker, J. (2021). *Unnerved: Anxiety, Social Change, and the Transformation of Modern Mental Health.* New York, NY: Columbia University Press.

Suris, A. Holiday, R. and North, C.S. (2016). The evolution of the classification of psychiatric disorder. National library of medicine. *Behavioral Sciences.* 6 (1): 5. https://www.ncbi.nlm.nih.gov/pmc/articles/PMC4810039/

Tweng, J. (2017) *The IGen: Why Today's Super-Connected Kids are Growing Up Less Rebellious, More Tolerant, Less Happy and Completely Unprepared for Adulthood.* p. 342. New York, NY: Atria, an imprint of Simon and Schuster.

Waters, E. (2010). *Crazy Like Use: The Globalization of the American Psyche.* New York, NY: The Free Press.

Whooley, O. (2014). Nosological reflections: The failure of the DSM-5 and the emergence of RDoC and the decontextualization of mental distress. *Society and Mental Health.* 4 (2): 92–110.

PART 2

Unpacking the Relationships Between Stress, Social Supports, and Mental Health

We all experience stress, though the sources of stress vary widely by social context. Remember, by social context we refer to the social conditions that shape our individual lives. Family, neighborhood, school, and work all shape our social roles and interactions with each other. Social inequality is a fundamental social condition, shaping where we live, go to school, work, and the number and types of stressors we will face. Anxiety is a normal response to stress and uncertainty, but an inability to control stress (which is linked to social position and status) leads to poorer mental health. The stress process model posits that social context and status inequalities produce stress, which place individuals at greater risk for mental health problems. Social supports can provide ways to cope with stress and thus can help buffer the effects of stress on mental health. At the same time, group membership can also increase an individual's vulnerability to stress. In Chapter 4, we review sociological theories about stress, describing the major sources of stress. Our social roles are an important source of stress, especially our work and family roles and our ability to balance competing role demands. We describe the stress process model and apply it to illustrate the impact of COVID-19 on our mental health. In Chapter 5, we examine the role of social relationships and social supports, with a consideration of the college environment and peer supports. We extend the discussion of social roles to describe how our roles shape our social identities. Our sense of "self" is developed through interactions with others, and we briefly review sociological ideas about the development of our social self. Those with a marginalized identity experience stigma, and we discuss sociological insights about the stigmatized identity of those labeled as "mentally ill." We conclude the chapter with a consideration of cultural variability in providing a supportive environment and return to the importance of peer supports for those living with mental health problems. In Chapter 6, we describe sociological theories about suicide, focusing on the importance of social integration as well as conflict. The increasing rates of youth suicide has been linked to the idea of contagion, where incidences of suicide can lead to more suicides among a given group. We describe the major social conditions associated with suicide and end with a discussion of suicide prevention.

Learning Resources

An excellent documentary to accompany Part II is *Stress: Portrait of a Killer*, produced by National Geographic and Stanford University. The documentary links biological to social conditions with descriptions of a wide range of research (field research on baboons, lab experiments, the Whitehall studies, focus group interviews) from diverse disciplines on stress. A Stanford University professor and MacArthur Genius, Robert Sapolsky, takes the viewer along with his family and contrasts his summers collecting biological and observational data from baboons in Africa with his hectic laboratory work at the University. Sapolsky makes the important point that our environments generate stress. In addition, his research points to the role of status hierarchy in produced stress and the negative biological outcomes of lower status positions. In an interesting natural experiment, one summer, the dominant male baboons in one of his study populations all died after consuming poisoned meat. The females took over and subsequently created a more egalitarian society. Other research points to efforts to reduce status hierarchies in the workplace.

Discuss the impact that stress has on our physical and mental health. How does our social status shape our experience of stress and anxiety? What role do social supports play in dealing the stressful circumstances that we cannot change? How can we change the social conditions that produce stress?

CHAPTER 4

The Stress Universe

A powerful metaphor coming from Wheaton and Montazer (2017) is the stress universe, which illustrates the complex array of stressors we face. Think about looking at the galaxy, and the visualization of a stress universe shows how the configuration of our stressors varies over time, place, and social position. Our stressors include major life events, chronic strains, trauma, discrimination, and daily hassles. Our social roles and work all produce stress. COVID-19 exacerbated many of these stressors. We also face an ever-increasing number of global stressors including climate change, violence, war, and immigration. Okay, so we are all so "stressed out." What do sociologists have to say about the sources of stress? In the 1960s, researchers focused on stressful events, now referred to as the life stress model, and in the 1970s, sociological ideas about stress began to include the role of social supports and coping mechanisms. Other theories focused on how social supports and coping can work to prevent or reduce stress. These ideas about the role of stress and social supports are now included in what we now refer to as the "stress process model" originally articulated by Leonard Pearlin. The stress process model has been further developed and refined by leading sociologists, many of them Pearlin's former graduate students and now themselves leading scholars in the Sociology of Mental Health (Aneshensel and Avison, 2015). Stress research crosses disciplinary boundaries, with entire interdisciplinary programs devoted to understanding stress. Stress is biological, psychological, and sociological with effects on physical and mental health.

Sources and Types of Stress

Let's begin with a definition of stress, which is any environmental, social, or internal demand that requires an individual to adjust his usual behavior. While there are numerous stressors, Pearlin identified two major types: stressful events and chronic stressors. Stressful events are marked by a specific time or place – perhaps an auto accident. Nonevents can also be stressful, think about missed graduation ceremonies amid COVID-19. Chronic stressors are ongoing stresses and are often related to social structures, and a stressful event can lead to chronic stress or strain. The auto accident can result in not only increased insurance rates and a number of daily hassles, it can also result in long-term physical injury and disability that is a chronic stressor. Not graduating from college (a nonevent) can lead to the chronic stress of status loss and unemployment. Graduating from college, while generally positive, may also result in the chronic stress of student debt or the inability to obtain a job in a tight labor market.

Other major life events include marriage and divorce – with marriage seen as generally positive and divorce generally negative. While most of us view marriage as a reflection of romantic love and commitment, this does not characterize cultures where marriages are prearranged. Likewise, divorce may also be a welcome end to a difficult relationship. Generally, divorce is stressful if it results in economic hardship, especially when women bear the burden of not only childcare but also lower financial stability. A major source of women's poverty is lower job status and unequal pay, but also the reality of single parenthood following separation or divorce.

An interesting case is the Maure people, where marriages are arranged, and divorce is often "a cause for joy" (New York Times June 4, 2023). Oudane, Mauritania, is located in the far Western region of Africa, just below Morocco. The country is 100% Muslim and divorce is common. The New York Times story cites a sociologist (Nejwa El Kettab) who has studied the historically matriarchal Maure people, where the experience of women is valued. However, as in many Muslim countries, most women are married young into prearranged marriages determined by their parents. At the same time, Maura is open and supportive of divorce, giving women the power to initiate a divorce and generally gain custody of children. In an odd twist, a divorced woman is seen as valuable and mostly divorced women remarry. Now, this may seem like an extreme cultural outlier, but it certainly points to the power of social context. While the divorce rate of Maure women is highest among younger women (the majority of whom had their first marriages by age 18), we can wonder about the experience of cultures where marriage is based on choice and generally occurs later in life, as does divorce. We do know remarriage (or finding a new partner) can reduce depression, but what about the effects of divorce versus widowhood where the loss of a partner was not a matter of choice?

In the United States, the divorce rate of those over the age of 50, referred to as grey divorce, has doubled from 1 in 10 in 1990 to 1 in 4 in 2010. Researchers asked if divorce was viewed as either a temporary crisis or a chronic strain, due to the loss of income and financial stability (Lin et al., 2019). The researchers used data from 1998 to 2014 Health and Retirement Study, which is a nationally representative cohort study. They found that for older adults, divorce is neither a crisis nor a chronic strain, and they propose an alternative theory, that of convalescence, or gradual adjustment and recovery from divorce. It takes older women longer to recover from divorce than men (4 years as opposed to 2), but they do recover. The researchers also found that the effects of widowhood on depression are stronger than those of divorce. Repartnering was equally beneficial for either the divorcee or the widow, though women are much less likely to repartner than men. This could be due to age disparities, where men prefer to marry younger women, or simply that older women who are financially secure no longer see the "need" to marry again and they may have their own well-established social support networks. Clearly, the effects of separation warrant further investigation, as well as among young people for whom romantic attachment and loss can be a significant source of mental health distress. In the following chapter, we will turn to consideration of relationship churning, which is especially relevant to college students who go through a number of relationships and breakups.

Moving beyond life events and nonevents, sociologists emphasize the role of chronic stressors, which are long-term and ongoing. The most important are status stressors, which are associated with our social position and social class and consequently affect our access to resources, opportunities, and life chances. As Deborah Carr notes in her excellent book, *Worried Sick: How Stress Hurts Us and How to Bounce Back*, stress is not distributed randomly, it reflects patterns of inequality with gender, race, social class, and age differences. Poverty, discrimination, unemployment, and poor health are all major sources of chronic strain. Chronic strains can lead to stress proliferation, where one source of chronic stress can lead to additional stressors, easily seen with the earlier examples of a car accident, failing to graduate from college, and quite often with divorce.

Contextual strains are another source of chronic stress; they are linked to where we are in terms of a given social environment. Think about your own neighborhood or community. Experiencing COVID-19 was very different if you lived in the middle of a major city than if you lived in a rural area. The urban and rural "context" shaped our experience of social isolation, the daily hassles of social distancing, mask mandates, and access to health care. If you lived in a rural area, you had access to outdoor space and did not need to be locked in your apartment or wear a mask to simply walk the dog. However, you may have lacked adequate internet access as well as the ready availability of takeaway food. You certainly had less access to health care with most rural areas having fewer hospitals and limited availability of mental health providers. While all hospitals were overwhelmed, rural hospitals generally lacked the capacity to treat patients and also suffered more severe workforce shortages.

Our roles define who we are and provide us with an important source of self-esteem and mastery. However, they can produce chronic stress or role strain, which includes role conflict, role overload, and unexpected role changes. Role conflict can occur when people disagree about the expectations of a given role. Think about your current role as a college student; how would you list your major "duties" as a student? Would parents or professors agree with your list of priorities? Students may view the role of college student as an opportunity to engage in new experiences and want to take a variety of "interesting" classes. Their parents may be more focused on a student selecting a major and earning a marketable degree. Professors expect students to attend class, to be attentive, and to prioritize study time and homework. Beyond that, professors have diverse standards, which can vary class to class and professor to professor.

Role conflict can also occur between diverse expectations of the student role, for example, coursework and study as opposed to involvement in student government, social clubs, and support for student athletics. Make a list of all the things you COULD be doing as a student, and another list of what you SHOULD be doing. Role overload occurs when we have simply too many things to do to fulfill a given role. What about if you also have to work? Role conflict occurs when we have two or more roles that produce conflicting demands.

Sometimes each of our conflicting roles also involve role overload. Trying to juggle the demands of work, family, and education produce stress, which can result in mental distress. An important outcome of college is learning how to juggle competing demands and to cope with stress in productive ways. That is the core of mastery, and college is one environment that encourages positive well-being by promoting learning, which involves mastery, which in turn reduces chronic strain.

A final concept relevant to the stress universe is that of stress contagion. The stressful experiences of others can affect our well-being – stress can travel through networks. The repeated refrain that we are all "stressed out" is certainly a result of stress proliferation, and the same can be said for anxiety as well. However, stress contagion is a major concern especially when considering younger people. Anxiety and depression have increased significantly for adolescents and young adults, as have rates of suicide. Data from a survey administered by the Centers for Disease Control and Prevention in 2021 found that 60% of teenage girls felt persistently sad or hopeless; one in three had considered suicide, with slightly over one in ten actually attempting suicide. A much higher number of youth who identified as LGBTQ+ had attempted suicide. We will return to the issue of suicide in Chapter 6, but the idea of contagion is important to preventing suicide. Adolescents and young adults are influenced by their peers, and news of suicide can increase the risk of suicidal ideation. In addition, information about "how to" successfully commit suicide via YouTube and social media has been hypothesized to lead to increased suicidal attempts. We will discuss suicide in a latter chapter, but stress contagion has certainly led to most of us feeling increasingly "stressed out" or "worried sick."

Work-related Stress

Work is a significant source of stress, so we turn to sociological insights on the relationship between work and stress. Prior to COVID-19, job-related stress was clearly linked to longer working hours and low pay, along with the degree of control a worker had over how to do his work. Job-related stress is also linked to the degree of control we have over our work, referred to as decision latitude (do we have power to make decisions) or skill discretion (we have the ability to control our work due to our unique skills and training). For example, nurses have a great deal of control due to their advanced skills, but they do not have as much decision-making power as do physicians. In addition, the degree to which work involves a high level of psychological demands from customers, clients, or co-workers is also a source of job-related stress. Nurses have high rates of job-related stress as they face demands from patients, families, and coworkers, but they have relatively less decision latitude and autonomy (compared to the physicians who oversee their work). In contrast, architects have a great deal of decision-making latitude and skill discretion and few psychological demands. Drawing on the extensive analysis of jobs and work by Karasek and Theorell (1990), those jobs most at risk for job-related mental distress are:

1. Low in control over work (tasks and decisions).
2. High in psychological demands.
3. Low in physical exertion.
4. Socially isolated from other workers.

These "high-strain" jobs were associated with higher rates of depression, exhaustion, absenteeism, and job dissatisfaction. Physical activity, or exertion, can help alleviate stress and distress, which can make a fairly low status job (for example delivery man or restaurant server) less stressful than the person stuck in their small, windowless office for hours day after day. Consider what type of job meets all of the criteria listed earlier. The person on the other end of a computer or phone taking our order, answering our questions, or solving our problem. While computers can bring increased challenges and opportunities for learning, the tasks may be monotonous, and computers can be used to monitor and control our work. Extensive time working with video display terminal leads to various health-related problems, including eye strain, headaches, and shoulder and back pain. A great deal of computer-assisted work is farmed out to Third World countries where there are fewer governmental restrictions over work hours and minimum standards for working conditions and pay. The exploitation of women and children is a global concern, and even in the United States, there is evidence of violations to child labor laws.

College students are often likely to work in high stress or strain jobs, but they know these jobs are temporary and may even provide valuable skills training, as well as learning how to work with a difficult boss, client, or customer. A significant source of stress is due to job insecurity, and computer technology and artificial intelligence clearly pose a threat to existing jobs. Concerns over work-related stress become critical when there are accumulated sources of job strain over time, where low pay, lack of control or mastery, and high levels of psychological demands converge.

In contrast, Karasek and Theorell (1990) identified the elements for nonstressful work environments. These job characteristics are very relevant to understanding the social context of work.

1. Equity: The feeling by workers that there is fairness and equity in the workplace.

2. Inclusion: Participation in decision-making processes.

3. Physical environment: There is the opportunity for physical activity, but not to excess. There are also few physical risks or health hazards, which include not only jobs that are dangerous but also jobs that involve working in environments that are noisy, dirty, or simply unpleasant.

4. Social interaction: Rather than being isolated, workers interact with each other, often in teams. There are respectful interactions between workers at all levels and relatively few layers of bureaucratic control and more participatory decision-making.

5. Feedback between workers and their customers is direct and allows for improvement and creativity.

A key source of stress is uncertainty, which can involve job insecurity and what sociologists have identified as precarious work (Kalleberg, 2009). Precarious work occurs when you have little control over your work schedule, and the times and hours you work are unpredictable or unstable. The rise in precarious work occurred with the transition from manufacturing jobs to the service economy, beginning in the 1970s and accelerated with the recession of 2007–2010. Manufacturing jobs involve production of goods, such as steel or automobiles while service jobs involve providing services to customers. Service jobs include those in retail, restaurants, hotels, banking, telecommunication, and health care. In terms of college programs, there has been growth in programs targeting hospitality, pointing to the professionalization of service sector work.

Other social and political trends also accelerated the rise of precarious employment. Along with the decline in manufacturing jobs, which was most evident in the 1970s–1980s with deindustrialization and extensive downsizing of even managerial jobs, there was decline in union membership. Unions helped blue collar workers negotiate pay, work hours, and benefits and these jobs were extremely stable. The service and professional sectors have been far less likely to be unionized, a factor in both lower wages and fewer benefits as well as precarious work. Welfare reform in the 1990s reduced the social safety net with restrictions on unemployment benefits, food stamps, and health coverage. At the same time, wages have not kept up with the cost of living. Many jobs in the service sector are part-time and do not provide benefits such as health insurance, compensation for work-related disability, or retirement. However, there have been a number of drives for unionization, for example, Starbucks and Amazon. There were several unionized strikes in 2023, including railroad workers, auto workers, and health care workers. Public support for unions is also increasing.

Another important trend has been the rise in single-parent families, with black women much more likely to the head of black households (18%) than white women (6%) of white households (United State Census Bureau 2022). Women must not only work to provide for their children, they also have to pay for childcare while they work. Service sector jobs are often low wage with unpredictable work schedules, making childcare a real challenge. Night shifts are especially problematic but are often required by jobs in the service sector, especially health care jobs. Minority single-parent households are most likely to experience poverty and must do multiple part-time jobs to meet expenses. For a single parent, juggling two jobs and childcare makes welfare benefits a sensible option; however, in addition to extensive bureaucratic barriers to benefits, there are often work requirements.

Juggling the demands of the job conflict with family responsibilities and other aspects of our lives, for example education or other meaningful social involvements, results in work–life conflict. The economic insecurity of precarious jobs and work–life conflict all reduce our overall well-being as well as our happiness (Schneider and Harknett, 2019). Well-being was assessed in this study as nonspecific distress (the K-6 measure described in Chapter 3), measured by how often in the past month you felt sad, restless, nervous, hopeless, overwhelmed, or that everything was an effort. These researchers also examined sleep quality and found unstable work schedules, especially working at night, reduced sleep quality, leading to increased levels of distress.

Mental Health America (*Mind the Workplace* 2017) has focused on workplace mental health, and in partnership with the Faas Foundation created an online survey and posted it on their website, inviting anyone to participate. While not a random sample, these data are important to understanding those who have concerns about their mental health or the mental health of their loved ones and are looking for more information. The Workplace Health Survey collected data from 17 140 employees across from diverse workplaces in the United States between June 2015 and March 2017.

In terms of work environments in the United States, the majority of those responding to the Workplace Health Survey felt their employers had "unrealistic workload expectations," and they perceived unfairness with unequal workload expectations. The majority also did not feel they were paid what they deserved, and that they had to deal with overly bureaucratic policies and felt "micromanaged." In terms of work–life conflict, 80% felt that the stress they experienced at work had a negative impact on their relationships with family and friends and 63% found work stress had a "significant impact" on their mental and behavioral health (i.e. substance use), with a similar percentage feeling lonely or isolated at work. Close to half (43%) found that they always or often had trouble concentrating at work. These are all important mental health outcomes and point to the importance of workplace context.

In addition to descriptive data, the Mental Health America study (2017) compared unhealthy and healthy work environments, and their findings concur with those of Karasak and Theorell's analysis of good and bad jobs as well as more recent research on precarious work (Schneider and Harknett, 2019). Healthy workplaces minimized bureaucratic controls and micromanaging, allowing for what sociologists refer to as discretion over work tasks. Supervisors tried to promote safe working conditions, equity, and a sense of fairness, as well as recognition of skill-based competencies. In addition to support from supervisors, healthy workplaces promoted positive relationships among coworkers. All of these factors reduced workplace stress and promoted well-being.

The key findings of US scholars are also reflected in the 2022 World Health Organization's (WHO) *World Mental Health Report: Transforming Mental Health for All*. Job insecurity, a lack of control, relational injustice, and a lack of social supports were all associated with mental health problems (MHPs). The WHO emphasized that all countries need to provide safe work environments that not only reduce stress but also promote mental health. Mental health has to be integrated into workplace policies and supervisors need to be trained. The guideline developed by the Department of Labor and Employment in the Philippines was used as an illustration. Employers are all required to implement mental health workplace policies that raise awareness, prevent stigma and discrimination, and promote work–life balance and healthy lifestyles. In addition, supports need to be provided to workers with MHPs. An important addition to the background provided by the WHO report is that many people work in the informal economy, where work is far more precarious, and people are not protected by regulations. Over 60% of the global workforce is in the informal economy. The informal economy is evident in the United States when we consider gig jobs and those who provide a variety of independent services, including food delivery, transportation, and even musicians with their crews during a concert season.

The Stress Process Model and COVID-19

Stress and anxiety have become our cultural mantra, why is that? What do you see as the major source of the feeling we are all stressed out? How can we break the stress cycle? Let's look to developments in the stress process model for some insights. The stress process model posits that social characteristics (gender, race/ethnicity, socioeconomic position, neighborhood disadvantage, and the degree of segregation/integration) directly influence exposures to stress, the social resources to deal with stress, and the personal resources to cope with stress. The social resources include social supports and network ties, while the personal resources include mastery, self-esteem, resilience, and mattering to others. Obviously, our personal resources for coping are influenced by our social relationships as well as our social positions and status. Exposure to stress in turn triggers social resources and personal resources for coping with stress. Exposure to stress, coping mechanisms, and social supports all have direct effects on mental health.

What we have learned in the last 50 years of research on the stress process is that it is vital to include multiple measures of stress. In the 1970s, life event scales were primarily used; researchers now include recent eventful stressors, daily hassles, chronic stress, lifetime trauma, role strains, contextual stress, and discrimination. It is also important to include multiple outcomes, including well-being, mental health disorder, psychological distress, and substance abuse problems. We provide an illustration of the stress process model applied to COVID-19.

The stress process model continues to undergo development as the "stress universe" is modified due to changes in our social context in response to social pressures, such as COVID-19, climate change, and increasing social inequality (Figure 4.1). These are all sources of structural strains that have global impacts. We can see COVID-19 as

Social and Cultural Factors

Inequality

Polarization

Stigma

Stressors

Life events: death, illness, economic shutdown
Chronic stressors: income loss, food insecurity
Daily hassles: mask mandates, misinformation
Chronic strains: discrimination, social isolation

Resources

Social supports: family, friends, social media
Coping strategies: new hobbies, pets, exercise
Personal resources: mastery, self-esteem, resilience

Mental Health

Positive: well-being, happiness, satisfaction,
personal and social growth, flourishing
Negative: depression, anxiety, mental distress,
suicidal ideation, self-stigma

FIGURE 4.1   The Stress Process Model Amid COVID-19

a stressful life event, but it subsequently required social distancing and isolation, leading to long-term chronic stress for a vast number of people across the world. The 2022 WHO *World Mental Health Report* describes the global impact that COVID-19 had on mental health and summarizes the many short- and long-term stressors people faced.

1. Stress from the physical health impact of COVID-19 infection and illness.
2. Stress from grief and loss of those who died from COVID-19.
3. Stress from physical distancing and quarantines.
4. Stress from unemployment and economic displacement.
5. Stress from false information and uncertainty.

In addition to these stressors, health care systems were also stretched beyond capacity and consequently people could not access adequate physical or mental health care. A sobering global experience was not being able to spend time with aging parents or grandparents, not being able to be with them in the hospital or nursing home, or when they died. Funeral services were also disrupted, with many locations (including New York City and Brazil) having to resort to mass burials.

Stress proliferation was certainly evident with COVID, with many getting sick, losing their lives, their jobs, and loved ones with the long-term effects of all of these many stressful "events." Once again, the many stressors associated with COVID-19 were not equally distributed. Women, minorities, essential workers, and those in lower social classes all experienced more stress and more negative outcomes with higher levels of mental distress. Young people have been especially hit hard by COVID-19. They lost loved ones; a telling statistic is that black children in the United States were more likely to lose their primary caregiver, often a grandparent or mother (Lemos, Sosa and Vallejo, 2022; Mays et al., 2022). Schooling was disrupted with many lacking access to online learning. Stay-at-home orders produced isolation and loneliness and placed many young people at risk for family violence and abuse, all well-known sources of mental distress. Women also suffered, both by virtue of their lower economic and social positions, as well as the additional stress of meeting the multiple needs of children at home and/or caring for sick friends and relatives, enhancing work–life conflicts.

A major source of uncertainty is death – generally viewed as a major life event. As humans we have awareness of the future, which will end in death, whether we like it or not. However, before our own death, we will all experience the deaths of our aging grandparents and parents, loved ones, and friends. We will also experience the tragic loss of life across the globe. In 2023, a train derailment in India led to 300 people dying and another 700 facing injuries. Flooding in Libya resulted in over 11 000 deaths, with 9000 missing. The war in Gaza has resulted in a horrific loss of life. An important aspect to dealing with death is whether it is anticipated or not, justified or not, or simply tragic. This collective "angst" and uncertainty is certainly an important source of anxiety and depression, as well as frustration and anger.

Increasing inequality and poverty has also fueled polarization, political violence, and conflict, which has resulted in significant declines in well-being as well as massive immigration. Climate change is producing more severe weather events such as floods, tornados, and hurricanes. These events clearly result in long-term chronic stress for individual families and communities with the economic impact going well beyond the event. All of these have required us to make adjustments, but more fundamentally, they are sources of uncertainty. Uncertainty is a major source of mental distress and underlies not only major life events but also our having to cope with the hassles of daily life, such as the loss of a car due to flooding.

Precarious work is based upon uncertainty over work, and COVID-19 substantially increased the number of workers in part-time, low-income work that was deemed essential, such as delivery people and fast-food workers. Health care workers during COVID also suffered increased job-related stress and burnout, especially nurses, and all health care workers faced high levels of psychological demands from their patients and their families. The WHO report notes that COVID resulted in high workloads with few organizational supports for health care workers. Health care workers were also at very high risk for contracting COVID-19, with many health care organizations unable to provide basic protective gear or even time off when sick. While health care workers have a fair degree of autonomy due to their professional degrees and expert specialized knowledge, they certainly experienced exacerbated burnout. Burnout originated in research on white collar professionals, including nurses and mental health providers as well as teachers. Burnout is linked to the psychological and emotional demands of patients, clients, and students, which resulted in emotional exhaustion, depersonalization or callousness, and feeling that the provider was not meeting their professional expectations. With COVID-19, burnout among health providers and teachers increased to epidemic levels, leading to workforce shortages.

Concluding Thoughts

Stress is an important source of mental distress, and it is created and shaped by our social context. Consequently, the treatment of MHPs cannot be directed solely at the individual; interventions must be aimed at reducing the structural conditions that result in increased exposure to stress, less mastery, and resiliency for disadvantaged and minority groups, or those with less power relative to the majority. Social position and relative power play important roles in access to those social resources that can both decrease vulnerability to stress and help anyone to cope with stress. In addition to describing sources of stress and social support, considerations of social context situate stress that accompanies social status (i.e. social class, gender, race, age, sexual orientation) as well as role occupancy (i.e. spouse, parent, worker). Social context defines not only the sources of stress but also the social relationships within which stress is developed and mitigated. Sociologists have contributed a great deal to our understanding of social support, which we know can minimize, or buffer, the effects of stress and also improve mental health. Social ties and supports provide a sense of belonging as well as concrete resources. While addressing the structural sources of stress is clearly necessary, improving access to social resources and supports can also improve mental health outcomes. In Chapter 5, we turn to social supports. It is not the stress, but how we respond to stress that influences our mental health.

Student Exercises

1. Tell your own stress proliferation story. Think about how stress is different for college students than the stress experienced by other young adults. How does age and context influence our experience of COVID-19?

2. Describe your most stressful job, or the most stressful job a family member or friend has held. Why was the job so stressful? In groups, discuss your "stressful job" descriptions. Select one of these jobs, and redesign that job so as to reduce stress. Then discuss the feasibility of making these job changes. As a follow-up, discuss your "ideal" job or career aspirations.

3. Apply the stress process model amid COVID (Figure 4.1) to two contrasting groups. By group you can refer to a given occupation or category of workers, a given demographic group (defined by gender, race or ethnicity, or age), or people in a similar place (nursing homes). You might consider interviewing an older family member if you do not remember much about COVID-19.

References

Aneshensel, C.S. and Avison, W.R. (2015). The stress process: An appreciation of Leonard I. Pearlin. *Society and Mental Health*. 5 (2): 67–85.

Carr, D. (2014). *Worried Sick: How Stress Hurts Us and How to Bounce Back*. Rutgers University Press.

Kalleberg, A. (2009). Precarious work: Employment relations in transition. *American Sociological Review*. 74 (1): 1–22.

Karasek and Theorell. (1990). *Healthy Work: Stress, Productivity, and the Reconstruction of Working Life*. New York, NY: Basic Books.

Lemos, D., Sosa, P. and Vallejo, E. (2022). Latinx race and ethnicity data gaps: The HACER campaign and a call to action. *American Journal of Public Health*. 112 (10): 1412–1415.

Lin, I.F., Brown, S.L., Wright, M.R. et al. (2019). Depressive symptoms following later life marital dissolution and subsequent repartnering. *Journal of Health and Social Behavior*. 60 (2): 153–168.

Mays, V.M., Cochran, S.D., Selemi, J.L. et al. (2022). The accumulation of disadvantage: Black children, adolescents, and COVID-19 data inequity. *American Journal of Public Health*. 112 (10): 1407–1411.

Schneider, D. and Harknett, K. (2019). Consequences of routine work-schedule instability for worker health and well-being. *American Sociological Review*. 84 (1): 82–114.

Wheaton, B. and Montazer, S. (2017). Studying stress in the twenty-first-century: An update of stress concepts and research. In: *The Handbook for the Study of Mental Health*, 3e (eds. T.L. Scheid and E.R. Wright), 180–206. Cambridge, UK: Cambridge University Press.

United States Census Bureau. (2022). Table MS1. Marital status of the population 15 years and older by sex, race, and Hispanic origin. https://www.census.gov/dataq/tables/MS1.

CHAPTER 5

Social Relationships and Social Supports

If we were not aware of how important social relationships and supports are to our mental health, COVID-19 and the experience of social distancing certainly was a wakeup call. Our connections to each and our social bonds constitute what we mean by social integration. As analyzed by Emile Durkheim in his classic study of suicide, social integration is a critical factor in explaining levels of suicide in a society. Durkheim also introduced the term "solidarity" to refer to the positive benefits of social integration on mental health. Solidarity and integration both refer to the ties that bind people together and provide for social supports. The degree of social integration is critical to mental health, and sociologists continue to focus on the relationship between social support and mental health. Social support is essentially about our relationships with others – who do we talk to, interact with, and rely upon? Fundamentally, social supports provide a sense of belonging and mattering to others. Positive and meaningful social relationships are a core feature of overall well-being as defined by the World Health Organization (WHO). Social supports are especially critical to those who are marginalized and face considerable stigma as a result, so in this chapter, we address the role of social support for people living with serious mental health problems (MHPs).

Social relationships are often shaped by our social positions and social roles, which constitute the social context of social support and mental health distress. Young children have their parent(s) and perhaps siblings and maybe a babysitter or nanny – or they are too often home alone or living with an abusive adult. Some children have a more extended family with perhaps grandparents, aunts or uncles, or stepparents and siblings. Children and their caregivers may have a set of neighbors they interact with who also provide support. Other children may live in dangerous neighborhoods with drive-by shootings and gang violence. When we go to school, our relationships grow to include teachers, classmates, cafeteria workers, and maybe the bus driver you see twice every day. As we progress through school, those social relationships continue to grow more complex with new types of interactions, roles, and social expectations. In short, our social relationships shape who we are, and in this chapter, we examine sociological theories about identity and also consider the stigmatized identity experience by those with serious MHPs. We also examine the role of the college environment in shaping our interactions with others. Social supports are important as they can not only help us cope with the diverse sources of stress we encounter but also provide a protective buffer against many forms of stress.

The Critical Role of Social Support

Social support has been studied across a number of disciplines, most notably psychology and sociology, which leads to a number of diverse definitions. It is a complex concept with multiple dimensions, and the meaning of social support can change over time and within different social contexts, just as does our experience of stress. However, the essence of social support is our social relationships and what these relationships provide for us. We begin by distinguishing between the structure of social relationships and the functions, or purposes they serve. Structure refers to the degree of social integration, or sense of community, or solidarity. Alternatively, we may also be socially isolated, which is another aspect of integration (or its lack thereof). Our social networks are another source of social relationships; we might look at our family, our friends, work colleagues, and membership in a wide variety of social groups – religious, volunteer, recreational, or political. While we can list our network ties, it is important to consider the functions of these relationships. Our family and friends may be a source of emotional support, letting us know we are cared for. Family and friends may also provide us with tangible or instrumental support, money or the loan of a car, or a place to stay. Alternatively, family or friends may also be a source of conflict. We also look to our social networks for information, which is a common use of social media, and can vastly expand our network connections.

It should be obvious that social support can also be both positive and negative, though we tend to emphasize the positive aspects of social support. While social media is an important form of social support, it can also have a negative effect on our mental health. A critical distinction is between our perceptions of social support, or perceived social support, which is not the same as the actual help we receive from others, referred to as received social support. Perceived social support has been consistently found to be more important than received social support to mental health, which is odd as one would think actually receiving support would be more important than the supports we "think" we can count on. While we do not fully understand why perceived social supports are more important than received supports, it may be the simple fact or feeling we do have someone to count on provides some relief. Also, not actually having to ask for help may reduce the negative aspects of social support. For example, we know we can ask a close family member or friend for help when we need it, but then we might feel guilty or indebted, or even ashamed. Just knowing the social support is there may be all we need to feel supported and to reduce the anxiety about the stressful situation we find ourselves in.

Many events that are considered stressful (such as divorce or unemployment) can also have negative impacts on social support by altering our social networks. Our networks shrink and we lose a sense of belonging. Young people are especially vulnerable to what sociologists refer to as relationship churning (Halpern-Meekin and Turney, 2023), with frequent breakups in dating relationships as well as churning through different jobs, or college majors. Relationship churning disrupts social networks, sometimes in a positive way, such as finding a new set of friends, but often they can also produce mental distress at the loss of what was once seen as a valued relationship. Ending a romantic relationship is always painful, and often we seek out new relationships to help us cope with that loss. More fundamentally, relationship churning introduces uncertainty to our daily lives and certainly constitutes not only a major stressor but also the disruption of social supports and relationship ties.

Peggy Thoits (2011) makes an important contribution to our understanding of how social supports can help buffer the effects of stress by distinguishing between everyday supports and stress-related supports, and also identifying who provides these supports. Everyday supports are cumulative throughout the life course and generally include family and close friends. Everyday supports can help reduce the occurrence of stressful events and also contribute to a sense of perceived supports, positive well-being, and self–esteem, which can all help alleviate the negative effects of stress. Family is generally an important source of everyday support and many of us can relate to calling our parents from college when things were not going well for us. With a romantic breakup, we lose what was once an important source of everyday social support, and we try to replace that sense of belonging and feeling important to someone else. However, also consider your expanding network of friends as you go from high school to college and then to graduate school or work. They may be an important source of stress-related social support. Your friends understand the stress of studying for mid-terms, or changing majors, or job demands. Stress-related social support is more focused and consists of problem-related supports (both emotional and instrumental), which do help with the effects of a stressful situation.

We also need to distinguish between two groups of supporters: significant others and similar others (Thoits, 2011). Family members or friends are significant others, but they may not be familiar with the source of the stress or stressor you are experiencing. While they can offer various forms of social support, their role in reducing the effects of the stressor may be limited. In contrast, similar others are those who have familiarity with the source of the stressor and can provide empathy, information, and advice. For example, during a divorce, one's significant others (family members) may not be empathic or understanding, though they can help with the financial impact of a divorce. Fellow divorcees or coworkers (similar others) may have more insight and empathy and will constitute a more concrete social support network. Peer supports build upon the experiences of sim-ilar others and can provide both everyday supports and stress-related supports, as we will see later in this chapter.

Stress can also have a negative impact on network ties and can result in a different kind of "churning" where our existing relationships can no longer provide continued assistance. Individuals with serious mental health or substance abuse issues often "churn" through their everyday social networks, exhausting key supports due to ongoing high levels of stress or trauma (McConnel and Perry, 2016). Family members may not be able to understand the experience of living with a serious MHP or feeling isolated and even suicidal. The experience of similar others, those also living with serious MHPs, can provide a more important form of social support as well as a feeling of social acceptance and belonging.

A final distinction is between bonding and bridging social ties. Bonding social ties occur when we feel a sense of belonging and integration within a given group, for example, our religious orientation or athletic team. Bonding ties can provide both every day and stress-related supports. Bridging ties connect people across diverse groups and can also provide both everyday and stress-related supports. In addition, both familiar and similar others can be sources of bonding as well as bridging ties.

We illustrate the complex nature of social supports with our study of those with serious MHP (Scheid and Smith, 2021). In this book, we examined The Oaks, a support group for people living with serious MHPs housed in a church. We found that shared participation in religious activities, or work in the community garden, provided an important source of belonging and security. These are bonding ties where individuals felt close to those with whom they shared an important connection. Bridging ties occurred when individuals went beyond the bonding ties of their local group to a wider network of people living with serious MHPs. In our study, we found that participation with the National Alliance on Mental Illness (NAMI) provides a path to advocacy and empowerment around efforts to reduce stigma. Bridging ties can expand our networks considerably and provide for additional educational or work-related connections.

Identity and Social Roles

An individual's social involvement and investment in meaningful role relationships clearly plays an important role in mental health. The key to the positive role played by multiple role identities is that we have different sources of satisfaction and opportunities to develop a sense of efficacy and mastery. Likewise, multiple roles provide additional opportunities for social support. For example, married people report consistently better mental health outcomes, primarily due to their higher levels of social and emotional support. Yet the quality of the relationship as well as the division of labor (both housework and paid work) and resolution of work life conflicts are important conditions that cannot be ignored. Work is also a source of a valued identity, providing for social status, mastery, and upward mobility. Our roles can expand our social support networks, providing increased opportunities for bonding and bridging ties. However, those with a marginalized identity face considerable sources of stigma and are often socially isolated.

More than other types of illness, mental illness fundamentally affects one's sense of identity – the question of "Who am I?" (Estroff, 1989). Attributions of irrational behavior (i.e. having a MHP) involves how we think; mood disorders target how we feel, and many believe that these thoughts and feelings are not "normal." The identity of a "mentally ill" person is a highly stigmatized and is a formidable barrier to resuming a "normal" life or recovery. As we learned from participants at The Oaks (Scheid and Smith, 2021), religious involvement can offset this stigmatized identity, providing a sense of being a "right" person, or a socially valued identity and a sense of belonging. Religion gave participants at The Oaks not only a place to go and a sense of belonging but also a valued social identity.

Sociologists have advanced our understanding of the relationship between identity and stigma by grounding who we are with our relationships with others, which is why we include this discussion of identity in this chapter. We start by explaining what sociologists mean by "self" or identity, and where it comes from, drawing primarily on the work of George Herbert Mead. Mead provided sociology with an interactionist account of selfhood, rooting the development of identity in our interactions with others. We only have a sense of "self" or who we are in terms of how others perceive us to be. Rather than a fixed structure, one's self is best understood as a process that is continually negotiated in the course of our interactions with others. We all have experienced that sense of dismay when we recall a self we once were (that bratty kid, the bully, the know it all, or the class clown), but what we do not always realize is that a particular "self" emerged in response to the expectations and perceptions of those around us at that time – be it parents, siblings, peers, coworkers, or significant others.

Mead defined the self in terms of its reflexive ability to be an object to itself; we can stand outside of our "selves" and see how others view and response to our actions. Often referred to as the mirror model of consciousness, or the looking glass self, we compare our self-imagination with our perceptions of how others see us and modify our presentation of that self accordingly. Self-awareness arises when we can conceive of ourselves as an object to another. This is termed reflexivity, and Mead argued it is developed in childhood during play and games where we learn to take the role of the generalized other. The generalized other is the "attitudes of the others who are involved in conduct" (Mead, 1934: 283) and internalization of the generalized other is a key component of our social self (Mead referred to this as the "Me" – the "who am I" we present to others). Mead used the example of a baseball game to illustrate the role of the generalized other. When playing baseball (or any game), you have to learn not only the rules of the game but also you need to understand the likely actions of the other "players" in order to know what actions you must take to "win" (or stay in) the game. The generalized other (part of our social self) is constituted by socially agreed-upon meanings, which arise out of actions that are shared and repeated by others in the course of our interactions. The generalized other is simply our understanding of what is socially acceptable behavior in any given situation. It is somewhat like Freud's use of the super-ego – it is societal expectations living inside our heads.

Many social theorists have conceptualized "mental illness" as the failure of the generalized other (Giddens, 1991; Laing, 1960; Rosenberg, 1992). Schizophrenia in particular is seen as the loss of the "me" self where the individual no longer shares the same inter-subjectively defined reality most people in society experience. It is for this reason that many sociologists define mental illness as violations of normatively defined expectations for thought and actions (see especially Scheffe, 1984). Those who are alleged to be "mentally ill" simply do not conform to social norms, or they act in ways that are inexplicable (incomprehensible) to us, as we discussed in Chapter 2. This is why recovery from MHPs is so often defined in terms of "normalization" – the objective is to live a "normal" life, the life we collectively define as "normal," generally by assuming appropriate social roles at a given stage of life. However, finding and fitting into "normal" social roles can be very difficult for those with serious MHPs.

As described by Goffman (1961), individuals with serious MHPs lack a viable self that is socially recognized and accepted – instead it is degraded, constituting what we refer to as a stigmatized identity. In order to be a person, the mental patient must accept the psychiatric view of themselves as a social failure, as one who must be fixed in some way, and what must be fixed is who we are (Goffman, 1961: 132). Goffman's account of the moral career of the psychiatric patient brings into sharp focus the way in which selfhood is constructed and reconstructed in accordance with the standards of a given social context, in his research, the reality of a living in an asylum.

Goffman also introduced key ideas about social stigma. We have known for some time that stigmatized beliefs act as self-fulfilling prophecies, with individuals living with serious MHPs feeling themselves less capable, which in turn results in social isolation, which then further reduces self-esteem, thereby increasing social marginalization. What we now understand more fully is the ways in which both self-stigma and social stigma interact to result in lower self-esteem and self-efficacy, lower levels of life satisfaction, and increased symptoms (Markowitz Angell and Greenberg, 2011). Our views of what others think are important to how we think about ourselves. Marcussen, Gallagher, and Ritter (2019), in their study of 156 adults in treatment in a community mental health center, found that acceptance of a stigmatized identity (my mental illness is a major part of who I am) was linked to poorer self-evaluation and greater distress. What is critical is that a growing body of research points to the importance of one's view of self as playing an integral role in recovery and identities that can counter (or resist) the stigma of mental illness are critical (Wright, 2012).

The Oaks provided participants with a place they could call home, where they were accepted on an equal footing, with a socially valued identity. Religion was central to access and acceptance at The Oaks, providing not only social bonds but also a sense of belonging. There were not many other places where participants felt on equal footing with others, or where they could fulfill normal roles. Participation in religious rituals and daily activities with staff created a special space of community solidarity. In addition, The Oaks offered important "bridges" to developing relationships outside of the program with another mental health organization. The National Alliance of Mental Illness is an important organization that not only links people living with serious MHPs to each other but also engages individuals in a wide variety of advocacy activities. These more formal social supports can provide a sense of empowerment and mastery so critical to not only personal well-being and self-esteem, but can also lead to resiliency.

Resilience is an important coping resource and is similar to mastery in that it can be influenced by our social experiences, relationships, and opportunities for growth. Much more sociological research needs to be done on the role of key social structures (especially school and work) in facilitating or reducing opportunities for resilience and positive coping among young people. More research is needed on how mental health delivery systems have responded to the many challenges produced by the traumatic stressors experienced worldwide by young people. We turn next to a consideration of the college environment and the role of social context enabling harmful coping mechanisms, as well as considering the importance of peer social supports.

The College Neighborhood

Colleges are close-knit communities with multiple sources of peer pressure and provide a classic example of the role of social context on mental health via the stress process model. Higher education is based on norms of status attainment and competition, think about how hard you worked to get into the college of your choice. Once accepted, students struggle to master new skills and competencies while also negotiating new friends and relationship and a high degree of freedom from supervision. Academic excellence is a prerequisite for future success, which produces a highly competitive culture with constant comparisons among students leading to high levels of stress and anxiety. Peer pressure provides for both stresses, as well as social supports, both positive and negative.

College drinking has long been perceived as a normative aspect of the college environment – an expected element of the college experience. The social context of college life, unsupervised weekend activities and parties, athletic programs and events, and expectations for community service have a significant impact on the norms surrounding college drinking. However, not all colleges are the same, and George Dowdall in his 2013 book *College Drinking* describes how each campus has its own culture with considerable variation in patterns of college drinking. What is unique about college drinking is that drinking begins and is reinforced among peer groups, and excessive drinking is an outcome of continued social support, illustrating how social supports can be both positive and negative. However, recent data (Monitoring the Future Survey on Drug Use 2021) show declines in college students who used alcohol in the past month (6% decrease) and significant declines in binge drinking from 32 to 24%. The lead investigator of the Monitoring the Future panel research (John Schulenberg) attributes the decline to COVID-19 and the simple fact that college students had fewer opportunities to drink with friends. However, the same data point to record high levels in daily use of marijuana, as well as increased use of hallucinogens (LSD and psilocybin mushrooms). Noncollege-aged youth had a slight decline in daily use of marijuana, although annual use was comparable to that of college students with historically high levels (43 and 44%, respectively).

What about the misuse of prescription drugs, such as opioids and stimulants, on college campuses? More and more students come to campus with a "diagnosis" of ADHD and in need of mental health accommodations to complete their coursework. College students have also grown up in a high school environment where taking a prescription pill is an acceptable aspect of our "pill for every ill" culture and many have been prescribed opioids for removal of their wisdom teeth. The ready availability of prescription drugs has led to reports of abuse. Synthetic opioids, such as fentanyl, are also available, which has led to a very disturbing increase in drug overdose deaths among teenagers and college students. However, the 2021 Monitoring the Future data show a decline in the nonmedical use of prescription drugs and opioids among teens and a significant decline in nonmedical use of amphetamines among college students, with rates remaining the same for noncollege youth.

If we look at patterns influencing the potential for future substance use among college students, the Monitoring Future 2021 data are encouraging, with declines in adolescent use of illicit drugs "the largest and most sweeping ever recording in the past 46 years" according to the December 15, 2021 report. Marijuana and alcohol use also declined as well as nonmedical use of opioids, tranquilizers, and amphetamines. This decline is also attributed to the pandemic, as adolescents simply lacked access to illicit drugs. However, the 2021 data show significant increases in a number of mental health indicators, with teens feeling depressed, anxious, angry, sad, lonely, and worried and having problems sleeping. Mental Health America also has data pointing to increased level of MHPs and has a number of initiatives to provide supports for Youth Mental Health, including a toolkit that can be downloaded for students of color as well as one for LGBTQ+ youth. However, drawing from what we know about the ways young people cope with stress, we need to anticipate that once college life returns to its pre-COVID-19 "normal," many students with unmet mental health needs will find solace in the comfort of drinking and getting high with friends in the relatively unsupervised campus environment. As of the fall of 2023, there are disturbing trends of fentanyl overdoses and deaths as many pills taken by students unknowingly contain fentanyl.

What can we do to make our college neighborhoods more supportive, or places for flourishing? The first and most obvious priority is to reduce competitive pressures for success, which are a primary source of stress. In addition, a trauma-informed approach is needed where ALL students have access to education, training, peer supports, and professional counseling when necessary. While most campuses provide counseling services, far too few counselors are trained in culturally competent care or sensitivity to the needs of marginalized students. Colleges must be proactive and work to meet the demand for counselors via expanded degree and internship programs. Colleges can also support peer-based mental health programs. Peer supports are critical as students are much more comfortable talking to other students, and a peer is more likely to be around when s/he/they is/are needed. Peer supports provide bonding ties with similar others, a sense of community or solidarity, help reduce stigma, and can promote a sense of normalcy. Peer supports can also be structured to serve the needs of culturally diverse students and can be integrated into academic programs and courses. Campuses can also involve students in advocacy training, empowering them to make needed changes in social systems and structures, starting with their campus environment.

Mental Health America has a number of initiatives to develop peer supports for young people (Box 5.1) following the empowerment movement, peer mental health support programs emphasize the "lived experience" of mental health challenges and provide opportunities for advocacy and leadership. Youth and young adults have shared the experience of COVID-19, online learning, social isolation, the threats of climate change, and the challenges of social justice movements that address not only racism but also homophobia and transphobia across the world. Youth and young adults also share

BOX 5.1 The MHA: A Comprehensive Approach to Youth Peer Support

1. Train all young people: General support skills, wellness, and education.
2. Go where people spend their time: School and community organizations, virtual, and text internet based.
3. Embed peers into all youth-serving systems: Mental health services, schools, and community organizations.

the experience of both positive and negative consequences of social interactions shaped by social media. "This distinct experience makes youth leadership and inclusion especially important, and youth must be viewed as an equal partner and leader in developing solutions" (MHA: *Youth and Young Adult Peer Support: Expanding Community-driven Mental Health Resources* 2022. p. 10). MHA provides online tools, training, and resources. This is a great way for students to develop practical skills and experience.

In April of 2023, MHA released a new report *Peer Support in College Mental Health Initiatives*, which was based on surveys and interviews with leaders and participants of college mental health peer support programs. The report provides specific information for college peer support programs to help them meet the mental health needs of a diverse student body. First, following the larger peer support movement, the lived experience of individuals is important to developing programs and enhancing leadership. Providing opportunities for the involvement of students from marginalized groups is especially critical. There are a variety of ways peer support programs operate on campus; some are student-led, others are led by staff (often through the counseling center), and others utilize collaborative models. Programs run by students were found to address a wider range of student needs than programs led by campus staff. A recent example is that students at UNC Chapel Hill have organized to provide drug testing strips and ready access to overdose medications, despite initial resistance from campus leaders.

A second recommendation is that peer supporters need comprehensive training, and students in peer support programs are interested in additional training. Campuses need to provide continuous education on mental health and the diverse needs of students. A third recommendation is to place a priority on trauma-informed and human rights approaches, especially in the face of a mental health crisis. For example, peer supports can receive training to help students develop "Wellness Recovery Action Plans" to promote wellness and response to a traumatic event. Another important issue has to do with student's mental health rights and the report provides a list of resources for students (for example, "Campus Mental Health: Know Your Rights" and "Model Policy for Colleges and Universities" from the Bazelon Center for Mental Health Law). Finally, peer support programs must be sustainable. That is that they need continued funding, educational resources, and opportunities to pursue a career in mental health. In short, peer support programs should be viewed as an integral part of the institution's educational mission. Collaboration between student leaders, peer support organizations, mental health professionals, and campus administrators is needed to develop and sustain comprehensive mental health supports for the campus community.

Cultural Variability in Supportive Environments

Social support also has important cultural sources, beginning with a distinction between individualistic and communal Societies. The United States is an individualist society, where the emphasis is on individual rights and autonomy. Communal societies emphasize collective values, placing the group ahead of the individual. Consequently, communal societies tend to have stronger family and kin supports, whereas individualist societies emphasize self-reliance and self-help. Individuals experiencing MHPs are reluctant to seek help from others and are more likely to seek out resources via social media or to self-medicate. In collectivist societies, there is less social isolation and a greater reliance on the family and surrounding community to assist with care. The distinction between individualistic and communal groups can be extended to diverse ethnic groups, towns, neighborhoods, and families, which is important to understanding social supports. Individualistic groups are less supportive and more likely to exclude marginalized individuals and communal groups being more supportive and likely to include marginalized individuals (Horwitz, 1982).

Globalization refers to a growing convergence among countries, with a general movement toward greater individualism following the dominance of capitalism (Grinker, 2021). However, there has been a great deal of more convergence in approaches to mental health that prioritize social supports. These include the growth in peer support groups, patient advocacy, an emphasis on lived experience, and programs devoted to recovery. All of these factors are addressed in the 2022 WHO report on Mental Health, which prioritizes community-based care as being evidence-based and effective in promoting recovery and human rights. Just as we saw with the MHA report on college students, the WHO recognizes that people with lived experience are a major force behind changes to mental health care quality and accessibility. Peer support services are about people using their own experiences to help others with MHPs and have been found to be effective for recovery worldwide.

The WHO 2022 *World Mental Health Report* describes a variety of types of peer supports, from self-help groups that meet face to face (even on park benches) to a peer-led, online therapy groups. One narrative from Dixoni in Tanzania illustrates her experience as a college student, which is similar to those of college students in the United States. She describes being in "soul pain" – with her emotions all over the place. Several friends committed suicide, and she tried it herself. She then started a new medication, began to see her college psychologist, and is doing better and living on her own. She attends a self-help peer group where she gets friendship and support. Like the members of The Oaks, she also has an interest in spirituality. In the end, she is "beginning to like herself."

Often a sense of community and belonging can be found in clubhouses for those with MHPs or psychiatric disabilities. Clubhouses and day programs provide people living with MHPs with a place to go to, and formal and informal social supports, which we saw with The Oaks. Formal programs seek to enhance concrete skills and empower individuals to live as independently as possible in the community. Informal supports are the sense of family and belonging, of having a home. One example identified in the WHO 2002 report that is found in over 30 countries is Fountain House. Fountain House originated in

New York City as a social club in 1948, which became the basis for a variety of clubhouse models that promote psychosocial rehabilitation. Fountain House clubhouses provide social support, not treatment per say. They have been found to be very effective in improving quality of life and meeting the goals of recovery as defined by the participants themselves. Members work with each other and staff to provide for basic needs (such as cooking lunch or gardening) as well as providing opportunities for members to enhance their own abilities and to meet their own goals for recovery (such as using a computer or art classes). Clubhouses can be designed to fit the needs of their members and can be focused around the special needs of a particular group (defined by their common age, ethnicity, religion, or community) and hence provide for social inclusion and empowerment.

Concluding Thoughts

While community social supports are clearly important, they are much harder to develop in individualistic societies. Another cross-cultural example is the Triest Model, developed in Triest Italy in the 1970s. This model replaced a mental hospital, moving patients and some of their nurses and staff to the town of Triest. The town was organized in terms of a social cooperative with the former patients providing essential services and many becoming self-sufficient. Well-being was enhanced not only for the patients but also for the staff that joined them. The Triest Model promotes social inclusion and civil rights for all mental health service users and has been championed by the WHO. Recently, the Triest Model was considered for use in San Francisco, and a review of the model along with barriers to its implementation is provided by Portacolone et al. (2015). The obstacles encountered in San Francisco point to the difficulties in fostering a supportive, inclusive community in an individualistic society. In the United States, community services are fragmented and reimbursement is based on medical necessity rather than on social services. However, the authors conclude that the "Trieste model has much to teach us and can serve as an important model of inspiration...it reminds us that mentally ill people are first and foremost human beings with social and economic rights... that their problems in many cases are aggravated by the society in which they live."

Student Exercises

1. Describe your social support networks. You might begin by identifying those who you are closest to, differentiating between friends and family. Then examine people you interact with on a regular basis, maybe through school or work. Differentiate between significant and similar others, as well as bonding and bridging ties. How did your social support network change when you entered college? In what ways do social supports influence your vulnerability to stress and in what ways do they buffer the effects of stress?

2. Students should access data from the "Monitoring the Future Project" or "The Healthy Minds Study" (or a similar data source in their own country or community) to assess trends in mental health and substance abuse over time. New data on social media and its relationship to mental health could also be assessed.

3. Students could access services at their college or university and identify ways to enhance peer supports for students with MHPs. Guidance is provided by various MHA webinars and reports (for example, in 2023, Dr. Scheid attending webinars and town halls on "Mental Health Disabilities on Campus," "Advocacy for Peer Supports," and an ongoing series for young people titled "Active Minds").

References

Dowdall, G.W. (2013). *College Drinking: Reframing a Social Problem/ Changing the Culture.* Sterling, VA: Stylus Publications.

Estroff, S.E. (1989). Self, identity, and subjective experiences of schizophrenia In: Search of the subject. *Schizophrenia Bulletin.* 15 (2): 189–196.

Giddens, A. (1991). *Modernity and Self-Identity: Self and Society in the Late Modern Age.* Stanford, CA: Stanford University Press.

Goffman, E. (1961). *Asylums: Essays on the Social Situation of Mental Patients.* New York: Doubleday Anchor Books.

Grinker, R.R. (2021). *Nobody's Normal: How Culture Created the Stigma of Mental Illness.* New York, NY: WW Norton and Company.

Halpern-Meekin, S. and Turney, K. (2023). Romantic unions and mental health: The role of relationship churning. *Journal of Health and Social Behavior.* 64 (2): 243–260.

Horwitz, A. (1982). *The Social Control of Mental Illness.* New York: Academic Press.

Laing, R.D. (1960). *The Divided Self.* New York: Pantheon Books.

Marcussen, K., Gallagher, M. and Ritter, C. (2019). Mental illness as stigmatized identity. *Society and Mental Health.* 9 (2): 211–227.

Markowitz, F.E., Angell, B. and Greenberg, J.S. (2011). Stigma, reflected appraisals, and recovery outcomes in mental illness. *Social Psychology Quarterly.* 74 (2): 144–165.

McConnell, W.R. and Perry, B.L. (2016). The revolving door: Patient needs and network turnover during mental health treatment. In: *50 Years After Deinstitutionalization: Mental Illness in Contemporary Communities. Advances in Medical Sociology,* (ed. B. Perry): 119–146. Howard House, UK: Emerald Publishing Limited.

Mead, G.H. (1934). *Mind, Self, and Society.* Chicago: University of Chicago Press.

Portacolone, E, Stevan P. S., Mezzina, R., Scheper-Hughes, N. and Okin R. L. (2015). *Culture of Medicine and Psychiatry.* doi 10.1007/s11013-015-9458-2.

Rosenberg, M. (1992). *The Unread Mind: Unraveling the Mystery of Madness.* New York: Lexington Books.

Scheffe, T. J. (1984). *Being Mentally Ill: A Sociological Theory.* New York: Aldine.

Scheid, T. L. and Smith, S. M. (2021). *Ties That Enable: Community Solidarity for People Living with Serious Mental Illness.* New Brunswick, NJ: Rutgers University Press.

Thoits, P. (2011). Mechanisms linking social ties and support to physical and mental health. *Journal of Health and Social Behavior.* 52 (2): 145–161.

Wright, A. G. (2012). Social defeat in recovery-oriented supported housing: Moral experience, stigma, and ideological resistance. *Culture of Medicine and Psychiatry.* 36: 660–678.

CHAPTER 6

Understanding Suicide and Prevention

Suicide is now a major leading cause of death for young people across the world, and the World Health Organization (WHO) has identified suicide prevention as an international priority. According to 2015 CDC data, in the United States, for every successful suicide there are 200 attempts, which is a frightening statistic. While men are more likely to die from suicide, the rates among women are increasing. Age is also significant, with younger adolescents having lower rates of suicide than the older groups (comparing three groups: 10–14; 15–19; 20–24), although rates are higher for all young people in rural areas. While mental distress is clearly a critical factor, younger people may be more adaptable, though they are more likely to feel helpless and to have fewer coping mechanisms. Suicide is related to social disadvantage. Young women and sexual minorities are at higher risk for suicide, but rates among young black men are increasing faster than for other groups.

Following COVID-19, suicide rates continued to increase for young people. Wong (2023) found that half of all college students had experienced suicidal ideation in their lives, with Asian American students having higher rates of suicidal ideation. Suicidal ideation is widely defined as thinking about or considering suicide, while a suicide attempt refers to nonfatal, self-directed harm. Suicide is a death caused by self-inflicted harm with the intent to die. It is likely that reports of suicide may underestimate actual suicidal behaviors. We will refer to suicidal behaviors as those that involve self-destruction, be they thoughts, actions, or death. This chapter examines the sociological contributions to our understanding of suicidal behaviors and identifies those social factors associated with suicide risk and those that can provide protection against risk. We then consider suicide prevention, providing general guidelines for best practices and ending with a consideration of the new 988 Suicide Hotline in the United States.

Sociological Approaches to Suicide

Emile Durkheim, one of the founding scholars of Sociology, is commonly cited for his contributions to the sociological understanding of suicide. However, what is less known is that Durkheim first published an article on suicide and then taught a yearlong course on suicide in 1889–90, before he began to collect the data on suicide for seven years that would result in his 1897 book, titled simply *Suicide: A Study in Sociology* (Lukes, 1973). A very close friend of Durkheim did commit suicide, and the topic of suicide had been a subject of much debate and was viewed as a growing social problem at that time with an unresolved dispute as to whether or not suicide was related to mental disorder (Lukes, 1973, p. 192). At the same time, Durkheim was interested in issues related to social integration given the current social and political divides in 19th century France, much as we have today. There was concern over "social dissolution" and critiques of excessive individualism.

Durkheim viewed suicide rate as a *social fact*, something that exists independent of the individual, and was interested in explaining rates of suicide, not individual instances of suicide. "He saw suicide as the antithesis of social solidarity, and a high suicide rate as an index of the inadequate effectiveness of social bonds" (Lukes, 1973, p. 206). This led Durkheim to differentiate between egoistic suicide (where individuals are isolated), altruistic suicide (where the individual is too strongly connected to society and commits suicide due to group pressure), and suicide as a result of anomie – where society does not offer social bonds or adequate regulation of the individual.

The difference between egoism and anomie is important, but easily missed. When one is isolated and lonely, suicide is possible – and this could be egoistic suicide or anomie depending on WHY an individual is socially isolated. Both involve normlessness, but egoism is a "breakdown of the self; anomie is the breakdown of the constraining legal and moral norms" (Lukes, 1973, p. 207). Suicides among white men following the 1929 stock market crash was a clear example of suicide due to anomie, the collapse of the economic framework, which was a source of self-esteem and mastery. In contrast, if an individual gambles and loses their savings and then commits suicide, that is an example of suicide due to egoism. A good example of altruistic suicide has to do with certain cults or military membership, for example, Japanese kamikaze pilots in WWII or the 9–11 terrorist attack in New York City where death was a certain result for the attackers.

In summary, for Durkheim, the most individual act (suicide) was linked to levels of social integration and dissolution. However, Durkheim clarified his explanation, excluding cases where "insanity may be considered a determining factor of suicide" (Lukes, 1973, p. 214). Lukes (1973) argues that Durkheim developed a social-psychological theory about the social conditions for individual health. The social "currents" generating suicide for Durkheim are relevant today, "excessive individualism, pessimistic currents, a state of crisis and perturbation… the state of deep disturbance from which all civilized societies are suffering" (Lukes, 1973, p. 214–5). Under adverse social conditions and inadequate social integration (or too much in the case of altruistic suicide), certain individuals respond by committing suicide.

Given the high rates of suicide we are now experiencing, there has been renewed interest in Durkheim's theories and research. While altruistic suicide is relatively rate, Abrutyn and Mueller (2016) reconceptualize altruistic suicide in terms of regulation, not self-sacrifice as Durkheim defined it. Regulation is linked to the broader cultural and social context, and high levels of regulation are indeed related to integration. Both regulation and integration can provide for "ontological security, a sense of a shared reality and solidarity, and a source of morality that gives purpose to live" (p. 62). However, too much regulation (or integration) can be dangerous. Abrutyn and Mueller identify three conditions that linked social integration to individual level regulation, which can promote the social conditions that result in increased levels of suicide.

1. When there are widescale social disruptions (or social changes) that rapidly break down existing social bonds and threaten an individual's source of identity.

2. Social conditions that increase the spread of harmful emotional ideas.

3. The unique ability to inflict self-harm.

This theoretically based article was published in 2016; before COVID-19 but following the 2008 recession and alarming increases in rates of suicide among younger people. COVID-19 has had an even greater disruptive impact, with economic dislocations, increased social inequality and poverty, political polarization, social isolation, and confusion over appropriate social roles or behaviors. Social media and disinformation increased the spread of harmful emotional ideas. Issues related to anorexia point to women's unique ability to inflict self-harm, long before cutting became common place. The widespread availability of guns has also contributed an individual's ability to inflict self-harm.

Suicide Contagion

Abrutyn and Mueller (2014) have also addressed suicidal contagion; that is, does having someone you know commit suicide result in higher susceptibility to suicidal thoughts? They first used longitudinal data to see if suicide attempts by a valued role model would result in suicidal ideas. Yes, there was evidence of contagion, with girls being more likely to be influenced by the loss of a family role model. However, when a friend had committed suicide, boys and girls were equally as likely to think about suicide. The loss of a valued friend also had a more lasting impact than the loss of a family member. Social relationships do matter, and if these relationships promoted a sense of alienation, or normlessness, suicidal ideation was more likely to result following a suicide.

These researchers then investigated a suicide cluster, a small suburban predominately white town with a high rate of suicides in their school (Abrutyn, Mueller, and Osborne, 2020). Suicide contagion involves a process of diffusion, where ideas are spread through groups and social relationships. A suicide cluster occurs when a number of suicides occur in one place over a short period of time.

For school-based suicide clusters, two suicides and one attempt constitute a cluster. However, in Poplar Grove (a pseudonym), there had been 16 suicides since 2005, with three occurring during the researchers' investigation. In-depth interviews and focus groups with students, parents, teachers, mental health workers, and young people were conducted to learn more about the community. In addition, an extensive media analysis examined how the media portrayed the suicides.

Two predominant "causes" were given for the suicides. First, they were a result of mental health problems (MHPs) or more generally psychological pain. A second theme was that young people were under a great deal of pressure, and this explanation become more widely accepted as the reason for why young people in THIS community were committing suicide. Another widely prevalent belief was that mental illness was stigmatizing, and that young people in this town were NOT mentally ill. Instead, young people were subject to too many high expectations for success, and suicide became an acceptable form of escape from these normative demands. Notable was that there were no efforts at suicide education or prevention, and the newspapers prioritized articles about social pressures and "buried" articles on mental illness.

Suicidal ideation was also found to be "normalized" in a study of Lesbian, Gay, and Bisexual youth (Canetto et al., 2021). The higher rates of suicidal ideation among sexual minority youth due to the acceptability of suicide as "an inevitable response to life problems" (p. 298). Not only was there greater empathy for those who committed suicide, but also they were seen as adjusted. Once again, MHPs were not seen as a primary source of suicidal ideation. Instead, it may be that the focus on the stigma and resulting discrimination and victimization "may contribute to the pathologizing" of sexual minority youth. Instead, attention needs to be placed on the contributions and advantages of sexual diversity to society.

Social Conflict as a Source of Suicide

While sociological approaches to suicide have emphasized social integration and our connections to each other, Manning (2020) identifies conflict as a major contextual factor behind suicidal behaviors.

Conflict need not involve outright physical fights or arguments (though they certainly involve conflict), but also "the clash between right and wrong" (p. 7). We can look to the current context of political polarization, racial conflict, and immigration as forms of conflict over what different groups perceive to be right. Avoidance of conflict is also important, which can result in suicidal behaviors as a form of escape, protest, or a cry for help. Conflict can also result in suicidal behaviors as a form of revenge, or punishment for those left behind. We can certainly see the role of conflict in considering the high rates of suicidal behavior among young people, be the source bullying, parental relationships, or unrealistically high academic expectations. Manning (2020, p. 95) makes the important point that suicidal behaviors may reflect our anger, or our own harsh judgments about ourselves. One of the young people in the PBS documentary *Hiding in Plain Sight* states that "self-blame is the root of suicide; you feel yourself to be a burden to others." High expectations (i.e. being the perfect student) can trigger harsh judgments in the face of the excellence of others and point to the power of social media to trigger feelings of inadequacy and lower self-worth.

Manning identifies social structures as critical to suicidal behaviors, referring to where we are located in social space. Major social changes, especially rapid ones, lead to more severe conflicts. As Collin in *Hiding in Plain Sight* describes it, "the world my generation is inheriting isn't pleasant, it's filled with toxicity." Competing cultural values, racism and discrimination, immigration, and the ravages of climate change all produce not just stress but exacerbate conflict between social groups. Globally, growing inequality and extreme poverty lead to a sense of despair and hopelessness.

Manning focuses on inequality as a source of conflict, and Durkheim also saw inequality as a source of social instability that would undercut solidarity and integration. The global economic crisis of 2008 (the Great Recession) resulted in greater downward mobility and rising suicide rates throughout Europe and the Americas (both North and South). In the United Kingdom, data collected by the Samaritans (a charity engaged in suicide prevention) noted higher rates of suicide among poorer groups, due to unemployment, housing insecurity, and other conditions attributed to lower socioeconomic position (Chandler, 2021). COVID-19 had an even greater global impact (see the PBS Documentary *The Virus That Shook the World*), and Manning makes the important and often-overlooked point that illness itself is a source of suicidal behavior. Cancer, disability, visual impairment, and the loss of the ability to carry on one's life all can result in depression and suicidal behavior.

Being in a lower status position puts one at greater risk of suicidal behavior. Manning (p. 41) does not describe bullying directly, but he argues that "being the target of insults, accusations, and punishment can trigger self-destruction." Sounds like bullying, and cyber bullying is often hidden from the view of parents and teachers. Parental conflict is also important to understanding suicidal behavior. Manning uses Western Samoa as an example where young people are expected to be subservient to their parents. However, with globalization, young people in Samoa are seeking greater independence from their parents, creating conflict. Consequently, 75% of the suicides among those aged 15–24 were the result of conflict with a parent. Manning reports similar patterns can be found in the United States, with youth in Latina families having higher rates of suicidal behavior following conflict with more traditional and controlling parental figures. Wong (2023) also identifies intergenerational conflict with parents as a source of suicidal behavior among Asian American college students, and Brossard (2018) found conflicts with parents and at school to be important social factors in understanding self-harm. Manning does not forget that the degree of closeness in a social relationship can influence the response to conflict. He (2020: 86) argues that "while strict hierarchy and harsh parental discipline increase the likelihood of a child's suicide, familial closeness means that milder degrees of discipline can invoke it as well." A decline in intimacy (or closeness) is also an important factor in suicidal behavior. Family therapy is one option, but most therapists and counselors can also teach young people skills to negotiate family conflicts.

Social Conditions Associated with Suicide

While stress and intense social pressure or normative demands are important to understanding suicide, MHPs also do play a role. Jamison (1999) provides a general treatment of suicide, drawing on research, literature, and firsthand accounts. Jamison is a psychiatrist living with bipolar disorder who has written eloquently of her own experiences. Depression and psychiatric illness are important, as is stress, and Jamison notes that stress affects not only our immune system, but also the sleep–wake cycle that can lead to exacerbation of symptoms for those with depression and bipolar disorder. Anxiety has the same effect, with racing thoughts keeping us awake too many nights. Increases in stressful life events play a role in the onset of depression, mania, and schizophrenic episodes and are also related to poorer relapse and longer recovery times.

Substance abuse is also predictive of suicide, especially when combined with MHPs (referred to as comorbidity). Depression, substance use, anxiety, irritability, restlessness, and features of the major personality disorders all lead to social isolation and to an "impoverished and solitary personal life" (Jamison, 1999, p. 111). A major framework for understanding the relationship between stress and MHPs (including substance abuse) is the stress–diathesis model. Stress interacts with the physical body, changing not only our immune system but also the chemistry of the hippocampus region, which also plays an important role in growth and resiliency. Chronic stress has the same negative effects on the brain as does aging.

However, we have to remember that stress is not randomly distributed; those in the lower social classes and minority groups all face greater chronic stressors. Gender and age are especially important, with young women at the highest risk for suicide, but rates among young black men show the greatest increases. The CDC's Youth Risk Behavior Survey collects data from schools and found suicide attempts rose by 73% for all black adolescents but rose by 122% for black adolescent boys between 1991 and 2017. In response, the Congressional Black Caucus created an emergency task force to examine the crisis of youth black suicide and to make recommendations (*Ring the Alarm: The Crisis in Black Youth Suicide in the United States, A Report to Congress from the Congressional Black Caucus*, Task Force Chair, Bonnie Watson Coleman). Young people of color face additional stressors related to prejudice, racism, and discrimination.

At the same time, racially ethnic youth may have higher rates of resiliency. Wong (2023, p. 23) defines resiliency as "determination, resolve, and persistence," which provide important coping strategies and life skills. While we tend to think of resiliency as a personal trait, it can be fostered within a community and increase over time as we age and successfully navigate life challenges. Resiliency can be modeled and fostered with programs and services that empower people to take control, even in the face of subordinate social positions. This is where peer groups and supports are important.

The availability and acceptance of guns is also an important social condition affecting the success of suicide attempts. In the United States, guns are responsible for the majority of suicides. While women are more likely to attempt suicide, men are more likely to die by suicide due to using more lethal means, such as a gun. In terms of prevention, limiting access to guns is important, as is adequate mental health and substance abuse treatment (both of which are currently lacking). Of interest is that doctors have very high rates of suicide, so reporting suicidal ideation to one's doctor may not result in adequate treatment. Jamison, writing in 1999 (p. 288), concludes that "major success at suicide prevention is (not) a realistic goal if treatment for mental illness remains out of reach for millions of Americans because health insurance is poor or non-existent." Jamison does a very nice job summarizing the many factors involved in how the stress–diathesis model helps us not only understand suicide, but also how to work to prevent suicide (Box 6.1).

BOX 6.1 Stress–Diathesis Model Applied to Suicide

Precipitating Factors:

Biological predisposition

Personality (temperamental factors such as aggressiveness and impulsivity)

Substance abuse

Chronic medical conditions

Social factors (especially trauma, isolation, chronic stressors)

Protective Factors (Social Supports):

Religion

Children

Financial security

Social supports

Triggers for Suicide:

Psychiatric illness

Drugs and alcohol

Personal or financial crisis

Other suicides

Suicide Prevention

The WHO (2022: xvii, Chapter 6) report identifies suicide prevention as an international priority, with the goal to reduce deaths from suicide (the suicide mortality rate) by one-third by 2030. The WHO has developed the LIVE LIFE approach that can be used by countries to help reduce suicides. LIVE LIFE is based on four interventions that have been found to be effective.

1. Limiting access to the means to commit suicide. For the United States, this involves guns; for many less developed countries, access to poisons (especially pesticides) is important.

2. Work with the media for responsible reporting of suicide. This involves not only addressing contagion, but also validating negative stereotypes about suicide victims.

3. Fostering social and emotional life skills in young people. This may be a strong sense of pride in one's identity, working against self-blame and guilt, and fostering resilience.

4. Early intervention, especially to deal with trauma and adverse childhood experiences.

In several sections of the 2022 WHO report, school-based social and emotional learning programs are targeted as necessary to mental health promotion and prevention, as well as suicide intervention. The 2022 WHO executive summary argues that school-based programs are the effective strategies "for countries at all income levels" and they provide many examples of how those bodies with responsibility for educational policies can move forward.

Researchers at the CDC draw on the 2002 IOM report "Reducing Suicide: A National Imperative" for strategies to prevent adolescent suicides (Crosby and Willis, 2017). Their recommendations are similar to those of the 2022 WHO report except for the addition of poverty reduction (Box 6.2).

BOX 6.2 Strategies to Prevent Adolescent Suicides

1. Universal prevention:
   a. Public education with school-based awareness and education.
   b. Media awareness
   c. Restrict access to lethal weapons (both guns and medications including aspirin)
   d. Poverty reduction
2. Community approaches: Communities that care, with efforts to deal with substance use as well as suicide prevention. Social media can be beneficial if used properly to provide education and linkages to social supports.
3. Implementation and dissemination of research and intervention efforts: A recent effort as an example of what Crosby and Willis mean is the American Psychological Association providing information to the NIMH on new research directions to prevent black youth suicide. Among the APA's recommendations was support for research on developmentally appropriate social media, research on the design, and delivery of school mental health services.

The American Public Health Association also provides guidance for suicide prevention efforts reported during the APHA 2000 meetings (Clinical Intervention. The Nation's Health. January 2021. Mark Marna "Health Workers Reaching Patients Who May Have Suicidal Thoughts") Given that many people who have attempted or died by suicide visited a healthcare provider in the proceeding weeks (according to NIMH data), there are opportunities for intervention. Healthcare professionals could use a screening method called QPR (question them about suicide; persuade them to seek/accept help; refer them to appropriate resources). Online training is provided by the QPR institute. Another resource is Project 2025, developed by the American Foundation for Suicide Prevention to reduce the annual US suicide rate by 20% in 2025.

Mental Health America (MHA) also has a focus on youth mental health and suicide. The report "*Young Peoples' Mental Health in 2020: Hope, Advocacy, and Action for the Future*" focuses on the need for leaders to "listen" to youth. Based upon their survey of more than 1900 participants aged 14–24 year, MHA reported that nearly half (45%) of those between 14 and 18 were *not* hopeful about the future (with more than half of LGBTQ+ teens not feeling hopeful). Those surveyed provided information about what resources they need and targeted access to mental health professionals and mental health breaks at work or school. They also wanted to learn more about mental health and training to support their peers' mental health. The report describes several programs that are supporting young peoples' mental health. Schools need to invest in peer support systems as well as mental health education and resources must also be invested in young peoples' advocacy so that they know how to make changes.

As a follow-up to the report, MHA has sponsored a series of webinars and town halls that are recorded and made available to participants. "Our Future in the Mind" was a two-day event held via YouTube (Friday evening and Saturday), which had several excellent sessions. The one on suicide featured a PhD psychologist (a black male) and three speakers who were suicide survivors. The survivors advised participants to watch out when people say they're "okay" – especially if they seem just a little bit off. Look for sudden mood changes, as well as dark jokes. It's OKAY to ask someone very directly if they are thinking about suicide, it helps to be "seen." Ask if they are thinking of hurting themselves; let them know you take this seriously. Take time to listen and be nonjudgmental. Often they feel alone and believe that no-one understands what they are feeling. Let them know you care with even small gifts of kindness. The theme of talking directly was reiterated by all the participants, and this is of course directly related to the stigma surrounding discussions of suicide or MHPs.

Another session was "Mental Health in the Schools" where participants described a number of initiatives in middle and high schools that incorporated mental health into the curriculum and promoted wellness practices. A simple thing is to provide a place where students can meet and discuss mental health, or just take a time out to "play." Youth advocates identified a major challenge that students are not educated about mental health or the political process and hence did not know how to make changes. In terms of college students, a community-based approach is needed where students have access to education, training, peer supports, and professional counseling when necessary, although there is a shortage of mental health counselors on most campuses. Some examples of what schools and colleges can provide include physical spaces to gather and talk; mental health days; care counselors (peer supports with mental health training), and training educators about mental health.

Faculty can also take an important role in changing the campus culture. Far too often, the message to students is that their GPA is more important than their well-being, that high levels of stress are normal, and that poor mental health is just the price you have to pay for academic success. This is certainly the message that high school students in Poplar Grove were getting, as well as reported by Wong (2022) in her study of Asian American college students. A supportive campus environment means increasing access to resources. It means teaching faculty to identify and assist students in crisis and to give grace when it's needed. It means institutionalizing peer-to-peer support networks, because students who are struggling are more likely to talk to other students. It means having a comprehensive suicide prevention plan and developing crisis response frameworks.

A major innovation in the United States is the Suicide and Crisis Lifeline (988), which is available 24 hours. Before the switch to the 988 Suicide and Crisis Lifeline, individuals with a mental health crisis would call 911. However, most law enforcement agencies were not properly equipped to handle these types of emergencies. Thus, oftentimes many callers did not receive any help. As reported in the American Medical Association in October 19, 2022 research on the 988 Suicide Lifeline has found that after speaking with a trained crisis counselor, most 988 callers are significantly more likely to feel less depressed, less suicidal, less overwhelmed and more hopeful.

The MHA held a webinar in July 2024 to mark the two-year anniversary of the 988 Suicide and Crisis Lifeline. The hotline involves collaboration with the Substance Abuse and Mental Health Services Administration, the MHA, and Vibrant Emotional Health that administers the hotline. So far the hotline has answered over 10 million calls, texts, or chats. The Biden–Harris administration has provided US$1.5 billion to subsidize and expand the network. In addition to expanding the network and improving georouting (routing calls to the nearest cell tower, not the area code), the MHA and SAMSHA want to improve upon data collection, both on who calls and the outcomes of the call. Confidentiality has limited data on even the race and ethnicity of those who call as well as follow-up, though questions about satisfaction about the encounter are asked at the end of the call. A major concern is whether enough trained staff can be found to respond to the increased demand for services. There are no specific educational requirements for those who man the call centers, but there is a 35–40-hour initial training and subsequent webinar training to address specific issues (for example, risk assessment or working with special groups). Current mental health workers are generally not able to devote a whole week to the required training. Another issue is dealing with burnout and high rates of turnover for a job that is emotionally demanding. Many states and counties have also developed their own lifelines to connect people to mental health supports, and the MHA is working to link all of these systems together as well as to improve access in rural areas. Other countries also have suicide prevention hotlines, including Argentina, China, and Uganda.

Concluding Thoughts

Sociologists have called attention to the role of social context in understanding suicide and the effects of inequality and disadvantage. Efforts by the WHO to prioritize suicide prevention globally are clearly important, and locating educational programs in schools and communities is a high priority. There is increased attention to the role of adverse childhood experiences (abuse, neglect, and trauma) in MHPs, self-harm, and suicidal ideation as well as the role of resiliency in dealing with adversity and disadvantage. However, there has been less attention to the cumulative effects of disadvantage and marginalization on mental health over the life course, especially for minorities. Chandler (2021) makes an excellent argument for the need for sociologists and health psychologists (and we would add public or community health workers) to work together to more fully understand the sources of suicidal behavior. More research is also needed on the efficacy of various prevention efforts as well as the role of schools in meeting the mental health needs of students.

In terms of a more sociological framing, peer and youth advocacy is an important source of empowerment and resiliency. Youth needs to take back the power to change those systems that are not serving their needs. Mental health is also an intersectionality issue and should be linked to efforts to promote diversity, equity, and inclusion. More open awareness of and programs to address mental health and suicide will also reduce both self- and societal level stigma. It is also important to simply be observant, especially for those at higher risk, such as LGBTQ+ people.

Class Exercises

1. Investigate how your school or campus is dealing with education about suicide prevention. What is your school or campus doing? What have you experienced? What is working? What isn't?

2. Examine youth suicide rates for your country or state (if in the United States). What social factors and context help explain variations in suicide rates between men and women, or for different racial/ethnic groups? Think about social norms, family structure, religious beliefs, as well as inequality and poverty.

3. Explore resources available for suicide prevention in your country or community and provide an assessment. Take part in a suicide prevention training.

Additional Resources

In the US Suicide and Crisis Lifeline 988 – available 24 hours
Website: https://988lifeline.org/?utm_source=google&utm_medium=web
  &utm_campaign=onebox
Youth: https://988lifeline.org/help-yourself/youth/

- Suicide is the second leading cause for the age range 10–24.

- Youth page has a break down on how to take care of yourself by asking for help, making a safety plan, losing relationships, and how love and friendship are about respect.

- How to help section – knowing the warning signs, listening, and supporting friends and loved ones.

- A list of resources for youth such as The Trevor Project, StopBulling. gov, among others.

Stories of hope and recovery:
Black Mental Health: https://988lifeline.org/help-yourself/black-mental-health/

- Only one in three black adults who need mental health care receives it.
- How to take care of yourself – make a safety plan, lean into community, ask for help, and limit your news consumption.
- How to help section – Ask and listen, be a support system for loved ones, and check in on them. Know the facts, mental health among black communities is not a one-size-fits-all approach. Care varies based on gender, age, ability, and location among other factors. Get them help and take care of yourself.
- A list of resources for black mental health such as AAKOMA Project and Center for Healing Racial Trauma among others.

References

Abrutyn, S. and Mueller, A.S. (2014). Are suicidal behaviors contagious in adolescents? Using longitudinal data to examine suicide suggestion. *American Sociological Review*. 79 (2): 211–227.

Abrutyn, S. and Mueller, A.S. (2016). When too much integration and regulation hurts: Reenvisioning Durkheim's altruistic suicide. *Society and Mental Health*. 6 (1) 56–71.

Abrutyn, S., Mueller, A.S. and Osborne, M. (2020). Rekeying cultural scripts for youth suicide: How social networks facilitate suicide diffusion and suicide clusters following suicide. *Society and Mental Health*. 10 (2): 112–135.

Brossard, B. (2018) *Why Do We Hurt Ourselves? Understanding Self-Harm in Social Life*, in English; French version published in 2014. Bloomington, IN: Indiana University Press.

Canetto, S.S., Antonellli, P., Ciccotti, A. et al. (2021). Suicide as normal: A lesbian, gay, and bisexual suicide script? *Crisis: The Journal of Crisis Intervention and Suicide Prevention*. 42 (4): 392–300.

Chandler, A. (2021). Socioeconomic inequalities of suicide: Sociological and psychological intersections. *European Journal of Social Theory*. 23 (1): 33–51.

Crosby, A. and Willis, L. (2017). Preventing adolescent suicidal behavior: Integrating sociology and public health (Chapter 25). In: *A Handbook for the study of Mental Health*, 3e (eds. T.L. Scheid and E.R. Wright). Cambridge: Cambridge University Press.

Jamison, K.R. (1999). *When Night Falls: Understanding Suicide*. New York, NY: Vintage Books.

Lukes, S. (1973). *Emile Durkheim: His Life and Work: A Historical and Critical Study*. New York, NY: Penguin Books.

Manning, J. (2020). *Suicide: The Social Causes of Self Destruction*. Charlottesville, VA: University of Virginia Press.

Wong, A. (2023). *Stories of Survival: The Paradox of Suicide Vulnerability and Resilience among Asian American College Students*. New York: NY: Oxford University Press.

PART 3

Structural Sources of Mental Distress

Social context refers to our social position in the social structures that surround us. Social structure is a broad term that encompasses diverse cultures, nations, religions, political frameworks, economic and educational systems, communities, and family arrangements. All of these structures shape our experiences of mental health. Social structures are also characterized by systems of social stratification, which is the ranking of social positions from low to high status. Social stratification results in varying degrees of social inequality and health disparities, with those in lower status positions generally experiencing poorer health, both physically and mentally.

Health lifestyles are shaped by our social and geographic contexts, including family, neighborhood, friends, and region (or country). Social class, race, and ethnicity are particularly important to health behaviors. However, our health lifestyle can change over the course of our lives, a concept referred to as a life course perspective. As children, our health behaviors are shaped by our parents or caretakers, with little choice as to diet and exercise. As our social roles expand, peers and coworkers are more important and our lifestyles can change significantly. Young adults are also more likely to engage in risky health behaviors. As we grow older, our health lifestyles become "locked in" and are harder to change.

COVID-19 increased health inequities globally, with marginalized and lower status groups experiencing a loss in economic position, poor health and death (morbidity and mortality), and increases in mental distress. The chapters in Part III examine the structural sources of mental health problems (MHPs), with Chapter 7 focusing on social stratification and inequality and the role of COVID-19 in increasing inequality. Our social class, or socioeconomic status (SES), is a major source of inequality. In addition, age, gender, race, and ethnicity are all sources of status differences, health disparities, and inequalities. In Chapter 8, we examine how diverse social statuses "intersect" and can amplify the mental health consequences of inequality and marginalized social statuses. Gender identity and sexual orientation are additional sources of social positionality that are important to young people, but are often viewed as deviant by the larger social environment. The stigma of mental health problems can intersect with other social status positions and lead to further marginalization, including homelessness, both topics which we examine in Chapter 9. We also include a consideration of stigma resistance as a source of not only empowerment but also social change.

Learning Resources

Students should view the last two episodes of the PBS Video: "Hiding in Plain Sight" (the first two episodes were used in Part I to explore the meaning of mental health and distress). The last two episodes directly address cultural diversity in expression and treatment of mental health problems for young people. The following quotes from the video provide for a good reflective writing exercise, but students can also develop an evaluation of the documentary in helping to understand the role of not only diversity but also of intersectionality and stigma.

> *"The world today is very different than the one our parents grew up in."*

> *"So much of what makes people sick has to do with where they live and are."*

> *"Time can erase the pain, but the child is forever changed."*

Stories from BIPOC youth and LGBTQ+ to illustrate stress and supports.

> *Trans: "It's a symptom of being marginalized by a society that does not accept us."*

> *Being Black: "Black people don't get to be mentally ill. The room for error in society is much narrower."*

> *Native American: "Trauma and Resilience are embedded in my DNA."*

CHAPTER 7

Social Inequality

In this chapter, we consider what sociologists refer to as the fundamental causes of mental health problems (MHPs). By fundamental causes, we go beyond the individual experience to examine the social contexts that place individuals at risk. Fundamental cause theory argues that individual risk factors (such as diet or exercise) need to be contextualized by examining the structural factors that place people at risk. Food deserts are a good example of how the social environment limits the ability of individuals to eat a healthy diet. Social class or socioeconomic status (SES), gender, and race/ethnicity are fundamental causes of disease that shape our exposure to chronic strains (such as poverty), as well as our resources to cope with chronic strains. These resources include economic, social, and cultural capital. Social relationships and supports also help us cope with our MHPs, but more importantly, they also influence our health behaviors and lifestyles.

Social inequality is a key feature of our social context and critical to understanding both the sources and outcomes of MHPs. One of the most persistent findings in sociology is the inverse relationship between social class and health, with those in the lower classes having poorer physical and mental health. These inequities are referred to as health disparities. Before we consider why this is so, we begin discussing what sociologists mean by social class or SES.

Socioeconomic Status

Sociologists generally use the term socioeconomic status because social class is a status characteristic, which defines our social position. SES is also preferable as the meaning of social class varies from group to group. Generally, income, occupation, and education are used to assess SES. In the United States and in many other Western societies, more education is believed to result in greater occupational opportunities and higher income, although this clearly is not always the case. In terms of social position or class, most people in the United States refer to themselves as "middle class" whatever their education, occupation, or income, which is another reason to use SES to refer to one's social position.

A useful understanding of SES is provided by Pierre Bourdieu, who distinguishes between three forms of capital, which define our social class position. Economic capital refers to material resources and is most closely associated with the role of income and wealth. Social capital refers more generally to our relationships, which includes our network of family, friends, and work-related associations. Cultural capital refers to our skills, habits, knowledge, and lifestyle and certainly includes health behaviors. In the United States, white collar and blue collar jobs may yield similar economic capital in terms of income and the ability acquire socially valued resources, such as a car or home. Social relationships are often enhanced by our education and work, and social media ties can also be a form of social capital. How many "likes" did your post receive? In terms of cultural capital, a white collar worker may prefer the symphony and fine wine, while a blue collar worker may prefer baseball and beer. New craft breweries and debates over the "blues" versus "jazz" show how diverse forms of cultural capital do not align neatly with ideas about social class. However, cultural capital is important to understanding health-related behaviors.

Health behaviors or health lifestyles are defined as the "constellation of health behaviors underpinned by group level identities and norms that are consequential for health and wellbeing" (Mollborn, Lawrence, and Onge, 2021: 388). Following Bourdieu, health behaviors are not simply our individual preferences but a product of our social relationships and cultural capital. Health lifestyles are cultural drivers of inequality, intertwined with issues related to class and race. We are prone to negatively evaluate the health behaviors of those who are from lower status cultural or social backgrounds, exhibiting ethnocentrism or a preference for our own cultural and class-based traditions. There are neither uniformly healthy nor unhealthy behaviors; we all exhibit a mix (i.e. we can eat a vegetarian diet and still drink too much wine with our dinner). However, we will be critical of behaviors we have been socialized to believe are unhealthy, for example, a pregnant woman drinking wine with dinner.

Health lifestyles exhibit both continuity and change over the life course. Children by and large do as their parents, so their initial health lifestyle is "acquired" or passed on. As children age, they develop more "agency" (having more control and autonomy) and often seek out new health behaviors and may "achieve" a new health lifestyle, often as a result of diverse social relationships or cultural norms. In terms of mental health, young people face a number of stressors related to family dynamics, educational demands, and peer interactions. As they age, they may draw upon various forms of cultural capital to deal with these stressors, patterning initial responses after those of their parents, and then learning new coping resources, such as exercise or mindfulness. Our earlier life conditions and behaviors influence our development, and as we age our health behaviors and lifestyle become more fixed and stagnant. It becomes harder to change health behaviors, including our responses to stress. Consequently, our cultural repertoire of health beliefs and practices are a powerful force in understanding sources of MHPs, as well as our responses to these problems.

SES and Mental Health

As noted earlier, it has been well established that lower SES is associated with poorer physical and mental health. It is certainly true that poorer physical health leads to poorer mental health. The experience of a chronic illness can result in depression and anxiety. However, higher rates of psychiatric diagnoses, especially schizophrenia, are also found in lower SES groups. This finding is also apparent in cross-cultural research, using a variety of measures for SES. Bruce Dohrenwend (1990) found that, in Israel, lower levels of education were associated with major DSM diagnoses including schizophrenia, depression, antisocial personality disorder, and substance abuse. One obvious explanation is that lower SES is associated with greater economic strain and resulting stress. Harvey Brenner in his 1973 book, *Mental Illness and the Economy*, analyzed historical data and found that economic downturns and unemployment were the most important sources of mental hospital admissions. This association had been stable for 127 years, with even greater impact (unemployment leading to more mental hospital admissions) in the recent decades. This study supports a tradition of which has found that MHPs have increased with urbanization and industrialization.

At the same time, it could be that mental hospitals are used to control, not treat, those with MHPs. Foucault (*Madness and Civilization* 1965) argued that "madness had become a problem, raising questions not raised before. At this time the mad had to be separated from other problems, i.e. the poor and criminals." John Sutton (1991) analyzed historical data from 1820 to 1930 and found that indeed, mental hospitals had more inmates than all other forms of custodial institutions combined, with the number of people being held in almshouses (poor houses) having declined. We will see a similar trend today with those with MHPs now being held in the criminal justice system. Social control is certainly a factor in the face of a lack of political policies to deal with inequality and poverty.

One explanation offered for the relationship between lower SES and poorer mental health is that those who have MHPs are more likely to "drift" down the SES ladder as they are unable to complete education or hold a job. This could be due to a basic lack of employable skills or to the greater stress experienced by those who are poor and unemployed. Lower SES individuals are also less likely to have access to health care, and may engage in unhealthy mental health coping strategies, for example drinking or drugs. We certainly see this argument offered in contemporary analysis of the "deaths of despair." Economic dislocation in the United States due to the 2008 recession led to higher rates of opioid addiction and drug overdose deaths, especially among working class men. As a historic example, the great depression of 1928 resulting in a high suicide rate for middle-class men. Both examples point to the loss of social position and status due to economic downturns.

Social causation theory is an alternative to ideas about social drift. With social causation, lower SES proceeds the experience of MHPs, rather than being a result of MHPs. Stress is still a critical mechanism, but individuals in upper SES groups also experience stress and have fewer mental health conditions and there is little evidence of them drifting from a position of privilege to one of poverty. While some individuals do indeed "drift" down to a lower SES position, the overwhelming evidence is that MHPs are a consequence (not a cause) of lower social class position.

If we look at sociological research on adolescents, we gain an understanding of social causation theory. Researchers conducted personal interviews with 877 adolescents in Los Angeles County (Aneshensel and Sucoff, 1996). Parental SES had a major impact on where children live and grow up, and they found that adolescents in lower SES households lived in neighborhoods with greater exposure to violent crime, shootings, gangs, drug use, and generally poor conditions. Exposure to these "hazards" led to poorer mental health, including depression, anxiety, and conduct or oppositional defiant disorder. Positive mental health was associated with greater social stability and cohesion.

In another study of the relationship between poverty and children's mental health, McLeod and Shanahan (1993) examined the effects of persistent poverty in the underclass. The underclass was originally termed by William Julius Wilson and refers to the mostly minority urban population with high rates of unemployment, women-headed households, and crime. While blacks and Hispanics had higher rates of current and persistent poverty, McLeod and Shanahan (1993) found little evidence of race or ethnic differences in the relationship between poverty and children's mental health. Poverty, not race, was the source of MHPs for minority children. However, recent research points to the influence of racism and discrimination on health. Villarosa (2023) describes that while she had always believed poverty was the source of health disparities, in fact structural racism plays an independent role leading to unequal treatment for middle and upper class minorities.

Structural conditions, including SES, poverty, and neighborhoods, also influence the types of psychosocial resources available to individuals. More recent research has linked SES to self-efficacy and mastery. Exposure to stress, discrimination, lower status jobs, and greater levels of parental, school-based, or work-related supervisory control all wear away self-efficacy and mastery. When stressors cannot be controlled, the belief in individual accountability can lead to self-blame for one's failure and harmful mental health effects. This is the negative side of more individualistic as opposed to communal societies or cultures. We will see that theories related to mastery are also important to understanding gender differences in the experience of MHPs.

Gender and Mental Health

Men and women exhibit different types of mental illness and disorder. Women have higher levels of mood disorder, anxiety, and depression. Men have higher rates of personality disorder and substance abuse. These differences occur globally as well, with depression and anxiety 50% more common in women (WHO, 2022, p. 43). From the late 1800s until very recently, women's higher levels of mood disorder were felt to be a result of either their hormones, or their more expressive, emotional personalities, as well as their greater propensity to seek out medical and psychiatric help. We now know that, in fact, women do experience higher levels of distress, linked to their minority status in most cultures and societies. Women experience more domestic abuse and childhood trauma, with long term mental health effects. They also assume more of the care-giving burden in their families, whether for children or aging parents, and often for both. Working women assume a greater share of household labor. These are all structural sources of stress and are related to culturally defined role expectations. Mothers can also experience postpartum depression, which often leads to psychosis. In January 2023, Lindsay Clancy strangled her three children and then jumped out of a second floor window, fracturing her spine (*New York Times* February 12, 2023). She had sought help for postpartum depression and suicidal thoughts and had been prescribed a variety of medications.

Men also face structural forms of stress in expectations, most often about work and economic responsibility for their families. Historically men have faced the significant stress of combat, an issue we see with images from the Russian invasion of Ukraine with men going into battle and women staying to protect their families. While the stressors may differ, what is more significant is that men and women respond to stress in different ways. Men are socialized to not express their emotions, which are seen in many cultures as a form of weakness or vulnerability. Consequently, men are less likely to discuss their feelings, less likely to seek help, and also less likely to be diagnosed with depression. Depression does not look the same in men; it often is displayed as physical symptoms including sleeplessness, fatigue, impotence, or physical pain. Anger is another response to emotional pain; women are more likely to channel anger inward with typical symptoms of depression, while men are more likely channel anger outward with increased substance abuse or combative behaviors.

An interesting historical contextualization of gender differences in mental health has to do with the identification of women's MHPs as nervousness due to their fragility as opposed to the "shell shock" experienced by men during WWI. As is nicely captured by the short story, *The Yellow Wallpaper*, women in the late 1800s displayed many symptoms of what we now call depression or anxiety, but which were characterized at the time as "hysteria" or "neurasthenia." Going back to the civil war, men also displayed similar symptoms of nervousness. During WWI the term "shell shock" emerged to explain the diverse symptoms men experienced given the trauma of combat. Grinker (2021) argues that hysteria and shell shock both represent psychological distress, though the manifestations were physical as there was yet no psychological language to describe depression or anxiety (Grinker, 2021). While women serving during WWI as nurses also displayed the symptoms of "shell shock", they were diagnosed with hysteria and discharged (p. 79). Grinker describes the effects of social class on diagnoses as well, with both women and men in the lower classes perceived as malingering and receiving more punitive treatments. It was not until the Vietnam War, and a recognition of the trauma of war, that the diagnosis of PTSD emerged, which encompasses the experiences of both men and women and crossed social and racial divides. Once again, we see the role of social construction in explaining the experience of emotional distress. Grinker (2021: 87–88) argues "the idioms of distress vary according to culture and history. One feeling, like anxiety, can at a certain place or time manifest itself through emotions like anger, fear, and sadness; in other contexts, anxiety presents as physical symptoms, such as a fast heart rate, shortness of breath, and dizziness."

Men and women respond to the stress in their lives in different ways, and their responses are shaped by diverse social and cultural contexts. Drawing on the theories of Emile Durkheim, Sharon Schwartz (1991) focuses on the social context of depression and differentiates between levels of integration and regulation. Altruism, a greater orientation to others and help giving, is associated with high levels of group integration while fatalism, a belief that one has little control, is associated with high degrees of regulation whereby others in fact do control an individual's choices and actions. Girls are socialized to be both other oriented and to accept strong normative controls over their behavior; the most obvious example is rules governing sexual behavior. A recent analysis of parenting among middle-class parents in two communities found that girls were subject to stronger normative control over their diets, which resulted in higher levels of stress and anxiety (Mollborn et al., 2021). These dual conditions of high integration and high regulation produce both altruism and fatalism, which results in lowered self-esteem in response to stress. Girls tend to be more dependent on others for self-worth and valuation, and thus more likely to feel helpless and powerless and to have lower self-esteem. Anger may also be turned inward, and all of these conditions are consistent with the etiology of depression (Schwartz, 1991).

Boys, on the other hand, are socialized in a context with less emphasis on group membership (low integration or egoism in Durkheim's terminology) as well as lower levels of normative regulation on behavior (or anomie). Consequently, boys and men are more likely to display antisocial behaviors in response to stress. That is, they are more likely to act out, to display aggressive or hostile behavior, or to resist normative authority and seek to actively break rules. An excellent PBS Documentary: *Men Get Depression* highlights the role of ethnicity and race in men's expression of different experiences of mental distress.

Schwartz (1991) refers to her theory as the norm hypothesis and contrasts it with the more traditional role stress hypothesis. Role stress theory explains the higher rates of depression among housewives by arguing that the single occupational role of housewife provided few sources of gratification and reward and was also relatively low skill and lacking in social prestige. Working wives experience higher levels of depression and stress because they are, by and large, working in jobs that are lower status as well as pay, and also had to face the conflicting role pressure of assuming responsibility for household labor as well as maintaining a job. Childrearing compounds these sources of stress. Depression among professional women is attributed to role strain and tension between professional obligations and aspirations and family commitments. Finally, the higher levels of depression among older women has been explained by their role loss; specifically the loss of family roles as children age. In sum, role stress theory argues that women experience higher levels of mental distress because of changing role expectation, produced higher levels of stress for which women were inadequately prepared.

Swartz's norm hypothesis encompasses various role stress explanations offered for women's higher levels of depression. However, Swartz provides an empirical test that contrasts the role stress and norm hypothesis by comparing the rates of mental disorder between traditional and modern Orthodox Jewish women. Both groups of women are subject to strong and clear cut normative expectations. However, modern Orthodox Jewish women live

BOX 7.1 The Importance of Social Context

Gender and Race Bias in Diagnosis of Anxiety

A recent study in the United States found that consistent with previous research, women have higher rates of symptoms of anxiety, and also have higher rates of a clinical diagnosis of anxiety. However, blacks have higher rates of anxiety symptoms compared to whites and Native Americans or Hispanics, but the lowest rates of a diagnosis of anxiety diagnosis. In support of sociological arguments about the importance of social context, Vandermiden and Esala (2019) found that individuals who experience violence, unsafe neighborhoods, poverty, and unstable housing are more likely to experience anxiety – but less likely to receive a diagnosis of anxiety, even controlling for access to care. What are the implications of these findings?

in communities characterized by changing gender roles with higher levels of professional work involvement. Role stress theory would predict that they would have the highest rates of MHPs, due to greater stress. However, traditional Jewish women had the highest rates of mental disorder. Their social context is characterized by high levels of altruism and fatalism, with value placed on self-sacrifice and commitment to others with severe limitations on expressions of anger (Box 7.1). That, it is not gender per say, but gender socialization into a particular cultural understanding of appropriate feminine or masculine behavior and role expectations, i.e. cultural capital, that is linked to mental health outcomes. Cultural norms about gender expectations are rapidly changing, throwing many of our cultural tropes into disarray, leading to confusion and stigma. We will address issues related to gender and sexual identity in the following chapter.

Race, Ethnicity, and Mental Health

Chronic stressors (poverty, unemployment, marital and family disruption, discrimination, and poor physical health) fall disproportionately on racial and ethnic minority groups. Part of this is due to the lower SES of many minority groups. In the United States, blacks are more likely to be lower SES due to the historical legacy of slavery and structural racism. It may seem long ago, but the Civil Rights Act was not passed until the 1960s. Members of other racial minority groups also face higher levels of stigma, as well as conflicting cultural messages as they are expected to conform to the values and standards of the dominant "white" culture. However, research has consistently found that blacks report either similar or lower levels of MHPs than non-Hispanic whites, both in terms of psychiatric diagnoses and symptoms of depression, even controlling for SES. The explanation for the "race paradox" that has been offered is that blacks have more extensive social support networks, including family ties, strong connections to a community, and religion, which have helped them to cope with the many stressors they face. In a recent article, Louie et al. (2021) find that blacks do have more family supports, higher levels self-esteem as well as religiosity. Likewise, Hispanics also have stronger family supports and community ties.

However, while rates of MHPs are similar, whites report higher levels of satisfaction and well-being. Researchers (Erving and Thomas 2018) examined emotional reliance, which is a negative psychosocial attribute where we rely on others for evaluations of our self-worth. Emotional reliance goes beyond asking "am I doing this right" to a feeling of inadequacy or lack of confidence in how to do something in the first place. Opposed to mastery, emotional reliance reflects powerlessness and is associated with those in lower status positions, including women and younger people. This makes sense, as you will tend to look to those in higher status positions for positive evaluations. However, emotional reliance has also been found to result in more MHPs, as it points to a lack of mastery, which is central to positive mental health. In their research, Erving and Thomas (2018) found that emotional reliance had a greater impact on depression, anxiety, and life satisfaction for blacks than for whites.

Racism and discrimination are significant sources of stress, and "Minority Stress Theory" includes discrimination as an important additional source of stress and MHPs. In a recent book, Linda Villarosa (2023) makes a compelling case that racism, not poverty, explains the poorer health of blacks. In light of recent attention to racial injustice, Moody et al. (2022) examined the effects of vicarious discrimination experienced by family and friends on distress. Vicarious discrimination was commonly experienced by black men and women with recognition of denied opportunities for advancement or employment among networks of family and friends, as well as concerns for safety amid widely publicized accounts of violence against black men. They found that black women experience greater vicarious discrimination, and they had higher levels of distress than black men. This study points to the need for more research on racism-related stress, which arises due to institutional racism, and is distinct from individual experience of discrimination. However, the effects of racism are also moderated by identity, with individuals for whom race (or ethnicity) is a central identity experiencing lower levels of distress due to perceived discrimination (Mossakowski, 2003; Stellers et al., 2003). A strong sense of racial identity is evidence of self-esteem and positive psychosocial resources.

There is a need for more research on the mental health experiences of minority youth who face significant stressors. The reality that black children are more likely to grow up in poverty, and in neighborhoods considered less than desirable has serious mental health implications. Erving and Thomas (2018) found that younger blacks in their study had higher rates of emotional reliance, which was linked to poorer mental health. At the same time, recent movements for racial justice may have created an important "buffer" in that youth in general are less likely to hold racist views and minority youth have a stronger sense of racial identity, leading to higher levels of self-esteem and lower levels of psychological distress. COVID-19 as a chronic traumatic stressor has had a significant impact with black and Latinx children who faced numerous challenges with family members working essential jobs and exposure to COVID-19, the loss of family members and care-takes, and struggling with on-line learning with limited access to the internet. Longitudinal research on the long term effects of the cumulation of multiple chronic stressors, commonly referred to as "weathering" for minority youth is clearly needed.

There is a growing literature on the mental health of immigrants (Takeuchi, 2016) and refugees (Goodkind et al., 2020). Stress proliferation is clearly an important process with immigrants and refugees experiencing the trauma of migration from often stressful social environments, the migration itself, and numerous stressors once they enter a new country. Post-migration economic stressors play a major role in mental distress, and the disruption of social roles and family relationships due to migration undercut usual sources of social support (Goodkind et al., 2020). There has been recent media attention to the mental health of immigrant children given policies for detainment and family separation. Children experience a wide variety of traumatic stressors pre and post immigration and family separation policies have led to unacceptably high levels of mental distress. While migration and immigrant status clearly constitute a chronic strain, foreign-born Hispanics have been found to have better mental health than native born Hispanics, despite their lower SES and educational attainment. In a recent study, Diaz and Nino (2019) examined whether family ties help explain this paradox and find that feeling close to one's family reduced the risk of depression and anxiety, but that having higher levels of family responsibility increased mental distress. We again see evidence for the important interaction between social roles, identity, and mental health outcomes. Immigration is a global issue, as is racial inequality, and there is clearly a need for more comparative research.

COVID-19 and the Mental Health Crisis

The COVID-19 pandemic exacerbated existing inequalities and led to a global mental health crisis, and should be seen as a syndemic, the synthesis of epidemics (Horton, 2021). In addition to the health pandemics of viral and chronic illness, the global context of systemic social and racial inequality, and what Simon and Mahoney (2022) identified an "infodemic," which includes not only the daily news stream and updates on COVID, but the overflow of disinformation leading to confusion and polarized views about protective health measures. All of these epidemics contributed to the mental health crisis and exacerbated existing structural inequalities.

Emerging in late 2019, by spring of 2020 most of the world had gone into lockdown with COVID restrictions leading to shutdowns, stay at a home orders and mask mandates, school closings, and a major economic downturn. The combination of economic distress and social isolation placed people at risk for MHPs as well as substance abuse. Older adults faced more severe physical consequences, including death, if they contracted COVID. With school closings, the lives of children and their parents were disrupted with increased levels of anxiety, depression, and substance use. In response to their

2021 mental health screenings, Mental Health America reported close to a 200% increase in the number of people seeking help for MHPs, compared to data collected in 2019. The numbers of those who screened "positive" for depression and anxiety had increased, with the highest rates among young people aged 11–17 with over 80% reporting moderate to severe depression or anxiety. In their 2023 report, *The State of Mental Health in America*, MHA utilized federal level data (not self-reports) and found that 59.8% of youth with major depression did not receive any treatment, with only 28% receiving consistent treatment.

Reports throughout 2020 and continuing into 2022 from various governmental and academic sources provided data that women, racial and ethnic minorities, and younger people suffered a "disproportionate" impact of COVID-19, including greater risk of contracting COVID, drying from COVID, and suffering MHPs. The 2021 MHA report on those completing a mental health screening in 2020 were younger (42% were 11–17), more likely to be women (75%), and minorities. The WHO's 2022 *World Mental Health Report* also documents the global impact of COVID, and the role of poverty, sexism, and racism on mental health. The WHO reports that "more than 80% of all people with mental illnesses live in lower and middle income countries" and describe the "vicious cycle of disadvantage which is linked to mental health" (Section 2.2.2). The WHO also addressed the diverse sources of social marginalization, including immigration, sexual minorities, and indigenous people, as important to understanding mental health as well as the lack of access to care. These various axis of status differences (stratification) interact in a complex manner to increase inequality and are also shaped by the cultural context within which people live.

Concluding Thoughts

We have very briefly addressed the primary social determinants of health: SES, age, gender, race, and/or ethnicity. An entire course could easily be devoted to each one of these fundamental causes. A key take away is that in order to reduce health disparities, we need to address social inequality. Public policies have to focus on the conditions that produce social inequalities, including issues related to wages and taxes for economic capital, enhanced family leave policies and education for social capital, and the recognition of the importance of cultural capital and knowledge in our current understandings of mental health. As we have seen, the mental health of minority groups (lower SES, women, racial, or ethnic minorities) is shaped by levels of mastery and control and viewed in terms of cultural stereotypes. Minority stress theory is an extension of the stress process model in that the experience of social disadvantage and having a minority status produce a unique set of stressors due to prejudice and discrimination. Critical is the sense of acceptance for one's identity as a minority as well as connections to others. Minority groups differ in the types of social support available and which they utilize, reflecting different types of both social and cultural capital. Their culturally derived health behaviors may be seen as inappropriate, and these negative evaluations are more likely when SES intersects with gender, race, or ethnicity. Age is also important in shaping our experience of health and health behavior. We turn to issues related to intersectionality in the following chapter.

Student Activities

1. Consider Schwartz's normative hypothesis and contrast the normative standards for boys and girls in your community. Are girls held to more rigid control over their behavior and appearance, friends, and leisure activities than boys? What about dating norms? Are there class or race differences? In what ways are appearance norms changing given the influence of social media?

2. Have students access recent data for a specific racial/ethnic group, focusing on understanding racial disparities in prevalence, diagnosis, and treatment of MHPs in minority communities. This is a good group exercise, with different groups each taking a specific group or population and sharing data with the class.

3. View the PBS 2021 *The Virus That Shook the World* (170 minutes, subtitled), which provides an excellent review of the global impact of COVID with a focus on inequality. Footage is intertwined with interviews and media accounts. As noted in the text, the examination of social class and racial inequality is very powerful, as well as attention to the role of the economic

and political context in dealing with COVID-19. Students can compare the experiences of families in different countries with their own experiences.

References

Aneshensel, C. S. and Sucoff, C. (1996). The neighborhood context of adolescent mental Health. *Journal of Health and Social Behavior.* 37 (4): 293–310.

Brenner, M.H. (1973). *Mental Illness and the Economy.* Cambridge, MA: Harvard University Press.

Diaz, C. J. and Nino, M. (2019). Familism and the hispanic health advantage: The role of immigrant status. *Journal of Health and Social Behavior.* 60 (3): 273–289.

Dohrenwend, B. P. (1990). Socioeconomic status (SES) and psychiatric disorders: Are the issues still compelling? *Social Psychiatry and Social Epidemiology.* 25 (1): 41–47.

Erving, C. L. and Thomas, C. S. (2018). Race, emotional reliance, and mental health *Society and Mental Health.* 8 (1): 69–83.

Foucault, M. (1965/1988). *Madness and Civilization: A History of Insanity in the Age of Reason.* New York: Vintage Books.

Goodkind, J., Ferrera, J., Lardier, D. et.al. (2020). A mixed methods study of the effects of post-migration economic stressors on the mental health of recently resettled refugees. *Society and Mental Health.* 11 (3): 217–235.

Grinker, R. R. (2021). *Nobody's Normal: How Culture Created the Stigma of Mental Illness.* New York: WW Norton.

Horton, R. (2021). *The COVID-19 Catastrophe: What's Gone Wrong and How to Stop it Happening Again.* London, UK: Polity Press.

Louie, P., Upenieks, L., Erving Christy L. et al. (2021). Do racial differences in coping resources explain the black-white paradox in mental health? a test of multiple mechanisms. *Society and Mental Health.* 11(1): 1–16.

McLeod, J. D. and Shanahan, M. J. (1993). Poverty, parenting, and children's mental health. *American Sociological Review.* 58 (3): 351–366.

Mollborn, S., Lawrence, E. M., and Saint Onge, J. M. (2021). Contributions and challenges in health lifestyles research. (2021). *Journal of Health and Social Behavior.* 52 (3): 388–403.

Mollborn, S., Rigles, B. and Pace, J. A. (2021). Healthier than just healthy: families transmitting health as culture capital. *Social Problems.* 68 (3): 574–590.

Moody, M. D., Thomas Tobin, C. S. and Erving, C. L. (2022). Vicarious experiences of major discrimination and psychological distress among black men and women. *Society and Mental Health.* 12 (3): 175–194.

Mossakowski, D. N. (2003). Coping with perceived discrimination: does ethnic identity protect mental health? *Journal of Health and Social Behavior.* 44 (3): 318–331.

Schwartz, S. (1991). Women and depression: a durkheimian perspective. *Social Science and Medicine.* 32 (2): 127–140.

Sellers, R. M., Caldwell, C. H. and Schmeel-Cone, K.H. (2003). Racial identity, racial discrimination, perceived stress, and psychological distress among African American youth. *Journal of Health and Social Behavior.* 43 (3): 302–317.

Simon, J., and Mahoney, R. (2022). *The Info-Demic: How Censorship and Lies Made the World Sicker and Less Safe.* New York: Columbia Global Reports.

Sutton, J. R. (1991). The political economy of madness: the expansion of the asylum in progressive America. *American Sociological Review.* 56: 665–678.

Takeuchi, D. T. (2016). Vintage wine in new bottles: infusing select ideas in the study of immigration, immigrants, and mental health. *Journal of Health and Social Behavior.* 57 (4): 423–435.

Vandermiden, J. and Esala, J. J. (2019). Beyond symptoms: Race and gender predict anxiety disorder diagnosis. *Society and Mental Health.* 9 (1): 111–125.

Villarosa, L. (2023). *Under the Skin: The Hidden Toll of Racism on Health in America.* New York: Penguin Random House LLC.

CHAPTER 8

Intersectionality and Mental Health

In this chapter, we address ideas about intersectionality, which refers to the reality that social status characteristics intersect. Intersectionality has its roots in black feminism, which called attention to how the fundamental causes of socioeconomic status (SES), race, and gender interact to influence the lives of black women. Sociologists have used the idea for some time to examine the multiplicative effects of social class, race, and gender. It is important to recognize that intersectionality can also apply to privileged status positions, contrasting the status of an upper class, white man with that of a lower class woman of color. There are many sources of difference in addition to SES, gender, and race including age, culture, ethnicity, and immigrant or native status. The term axis of inequality (or stratification) is often used to refer to the broad range of status differences in any given society or community. Intersectionality has expanded to becoming a primary framework for public health and is core to understanding the many ways in which intersectionality influences health-related outcomes (Bowleg, 2012). In this chapter, we address the impact of intersectionality of SES, gender, and race on mental health. We also address intersectionality in understanding the mental health problems (MHPs) faced by sexual and gender minorities as well as for indigenous people, limiting our discussion to young people. In addition to racism and sexism, indigenous people have experienced the exploitation of colonization, where they were displaced from their homelands.

Intersecting Social Statuses

Social class, gender, race, and ethnicity are interrelated in a complex manner with multiple feedback loops. Intersectionality begins with the idea that we have social identities that are multiple and interlocking and provides a "framework for understanding how multiple social identities intersect at the micro level of experience to reflect interlocking systems of power and privilege" (Bowleg 2012; 1267). In terms of identity, we are not just male or female, but upper, middle, or lower class, white, black, or brown, with numerous ethnic identities and cultural backgrounds. The interlocking systems refer to racism, sexism, and structural inequality, which also intersect. Female and black are two social statuses that are socially devalued, and African American women are more likely to live in poverty than white women. African American women also face demanding social networks, which may be an additional source of stress, rather than a coping resource. Keith and Brown (2017) provide a theoretical model for understanding how these intersecting social statuses affect the mental health of African American women, which emphasized the complex inter-relationship between race, gender, and social class. Mental well-being is influenced by not only the primary social statues of race, gender, and SES but also other social, cultural, and psychological factors as well as physical health and health beliefs and behaviors.

We begin with the inter-relationships between race, gender, and SES. African American women are more likely to live in poverty than white women; their educational attainment is lower, and they are more likely to hold lower status occupations, with lower incomes and fewer opportunities for mastery or control. African American women are also more likely to be unemployed or to work only part time. If we just focus on health care occupations, minority women are more likely to be found in lower status positions in hospitals or nursing homes, and to have more variable work schedules. African American women are also more likely to be single mothers, complicating their lives with juggling work and family responsibilities. It should come as no surprise that minority women suffered the most from COVID, due to the nature of their jobs, exposure to COVID, and attempting to parent children at home struggling with lockdowns. African American women are also more likely to live in disadvantaged neighborhoods, with fewer playgrounds, walking spaces, or access to healthy food. The PBS documentary *The Virus That Shook the World* does a great job contrasting the experiences of a minority family in New York City with a poor family in Brazil with a more advantaged family in France, contrasting living space and neighborhoods amid shutdowns.

Physical health is another important source of poor mental health. African American women have poorer physical health with greater risk of obesity, hypertension, diabetes, and heart disease. However, they are less likely to smoke, drink, or use drugs. Given less access to health care (due to either lack of insurance or a lack of time or money or transportation to go to a health care facility), African American women have higher death rates, with serious physical health problems often going untreated. COVID infection is another obvious source of poor health. The jobs held by minority women (and men) often placed them at higher risk for COVID infection, yet they were less able to access health care or vaccinations to prevent infection.

COVID reduces the immune response of the body, so the likelihood of subsequent illness and "long COVID" is enhanced. In her own experience of chronic illness, Megan O'Rourke (2022) saw nine medical providers and found that "despite being a privileged white woman … there are class, race, and language barriers to care" (pp. 60–61). With COVID, chronic illness and autoimmune disorders are "rising to epidemic rates" (p. 5). We are not sure how long the COVID virus will pose a major health risk, how it will mutate, or move around, or its response to vaccines or other illnesses. However, it is certain to decrease our overall well-being, ability to work, and lead to as yet poorly understood mental health challenges.

The cumulative effect of multiple chronic stressors results in higher levels of psychological distress, major depression, phobia, PTSD, and schizophrenia in minority women (Keith and Brown, 2017). Protective factors (which reduce the impact of chronic stressors on mental health) include sources of social support: marriage, religious involvement, and social participation. However, these various forms of social support were not available during COVID-19, increasing the cumulative disadvantages of being female, minority, a single parent, and having competing work demands. Keith and Brown (2017) also raise questions about how African women deal with their experiences of racism, sexism, and discrimination. In *The Virus That Shook the World*, the female-headed black family participates in a racial protest and is confronted by law enforcement with videos of the mother becoming separated from her teenaged daughter. At the same time, their resistance was experienced as empowering by both mother and daughter.

In addition to social class, gender, race, and ethnicity, social position is also structured by age and changing social roles. Researchers have found that mental health and distress vary across the life course with younger and older individuals experiencing higher levels of mental distress and those in their middle years having the highest levels of mental well-being. Levels of control or mastery provide an answer: younger people face a great deal of uncertainty as they navigate education, jobs, and relationships. In response to the stressors of childhood and adolescence, young people can exhibit externalizing behaviors that are more aggressive or internalizing behaviors such as withdrawal and gender socialization can play a role. Older adults face the loss of social status due to retirement, poorer physical health, and loss of social relationships. Adults in their middle years are at their "peak" in terms of career, income, and family stability. However, many middle-aged parents find themselves "sandwiched" between raising their own children and caring for their aging parents, with a greater burden falling on women as the caretakers in the family.

In terms of COVID-19, in a cross-national study, Na et al. (2022) found that while older adults had relatively high levels of mortality (i.e. more likely to die from COVID), they had lower levels of distress and loneliness and higher levels of resilience and coping mechanisms. Younger adults (18–34) had the highest levels of mental distress and loneliness as well as the lowest resilience and more maladaptive coping. Resilience is an important coping resource, and the authors suggest that resilience is not a personal trait as their analysis found resilience increased with age. Resilience may be similar to mastery; it can be influenced by our social experiences, relationships, and opportunities for growth. Much more sociological research needs to be done on the role of key social structures, especially school and work, in facilitating or reducing opportunities for resilience and positive coping. More research is needed on how mental health delivery systems have responded to the many challenges produced by the traumatic stressors experienced worldwide by young people.

Young People and Intersecting Identities

COVID-19 exacerbated the MHPs faced by young people, who can be considered to be a distinct minority group due to their overall lower status and lack of autonomy. We can use the term "adultism" to refer to the prioritizing of adulthood. Parents and teachers hold a great deal of power over young people, who often lack permission to make their own decisions, whether right or wrong. While we all faced increased anxiety and depression amid COVID-19, young people reported in numerous surveys the highest levels of loneliness, anxiety, and feelings of sadness and hopelessness. The CDC reported that emergency room visits for young people aged 12–17 increased by 31% at the beginning of the pandemic (MHA 2021, "Young People's Mental Health"). However, COVID had an even greater impact on youth who are black, indigenous, and people of color (BIPOC) as well as lesbian, gay, bisexual, transgender (including nonbinary) and other queer-identified youth (LGBTQ+). BIPOC and LGBTQ+ are two additional sources of marginality, intersecting with both gender and SES.

Proceeding COVID-19, rates of poor mental health and suicidal ideation were already alarming high for BIPOC youth, with men experiencing the greatest increases in MHPs. The CDC's Youth Risk Behavior Survey found that suicide attempts for black adolescents had risen by 73% between 1991 and 2017, with men more likely to experience some injury pointing to use of guns in their suicide attempts. Rates of drug overdose death, including both prescription and nonprescription drugs, also rose sharply. The CDC July 2022 Morbidity and Mortality Weekly Report showed an increase of 86% in drug overdose deaths for blacks aged 15–24 between 2019 and 2020. These high rates of increase reflect that rates of suicide and drug overdose deaths had been relatively low for young black men, so an increase from 5% to 20% will reflect over a 200% increase. In 2023, provisional data from the CDC show decreasing rates of suicide and drug overdose deaths from fentanyl, but rates for younger black men are still of concern.

If we examine self-reported data from those aged 11–17 using 2020 MHA Screening data (MHA 2021), we find some interesting differences in the sources of their MHPs. Overall, 72% of young people identified loneliness and social isolation, 65% identified social life or relationships, and 42% identified past trauma as the main source of their mental distress. However, there were some interesting racial differences in the ranking of the main source of their mental distress. White youth were most likely to select the coronavirus; black youth were more likely to identify financial problems; Hispanic or Latinx to select loneliness or isolation; Native Americans selected grief or loss as well as past trauma. Asian Americans or Pacific Islanders were as likely to identify social life or relationships as well as loneliness as the main source of distress (and these are clearly linked) while those who identified as more than one race were most likely to select current events.

In addition to the pandemic, BIPOC also faced growing evidence of racism with an increasing politicized environment. Black Lives Matter and protests in response to police violence against blacks, increased anti-Asian rhetoric, and associations of Hispanics as illegal immigrants all contributed to considerable mental distress and anxiety. Blacks were most likely to include racism as one of their top three concerns (19%), following by those identifying as more than one race (12%) with 9% of other racial/ethnic groups identifying racism. Asian and white youth were much less likely to identify racism as a central concern (MHA 2021).

Indigenous people across the world face an additional source of social marginalization and racism. Indigenous people (i.e. those who self-define as indigenous and belong to a community that experienced colonialism) inhabit over 90 countries and Paradies (2016) summarizes research on the impacts of racism on their mental and physical health. In terms of mental health, indigenous people experience the "colonial context of ongoing oppression, cultural, and historic loss, high rates of victimization and exposure to violence, poverty and other daily and chronic stressors" (Goodkind et al., 2015: 486), all of which lead to high rates of mental distress. Blacks, Native Americans, and many Hispanic or Latinx groups have also experienced the legacy of slavery or colonization. The historical trauma can result in intergenerational trauma, where emotional trauma can pass from one generation to another. This trauma can be expressed as anger over what was lost, or a sense of loss or hopelessness. For young people, trauma can result in higher rates of interpersonal conflict and behavioral problems, substance misuse, depression, and suicide. Goodkind et al. (2015) found that the 14 young Native Americans (aged 15–24) they interviewed experienced a great deal of anger and were disciplined or referred to therapy for anger management. At the same time, they expressed a strong connection to the land, which was utilized in building a sense of spirituality that improved interactions with parents and family members. As with other indigenous people, place and space are critical to a sense of well-being, given the historical displacement from tribal lands.

LGBTQ+ and Gender Diversity

An additional axis of identity is that of sexual orientation. Lesbian, gay, bisexual, transgender, queer, and other (LGBTQ+) students face a higher risk than their cisgender, heterosexual peers of experiencing symptoms of not only poor mental health but also poor sexual health (STDs) and sexual violence. Young people who identify as LGBTQ+ faced unique stressors and even greater social isolation and loneliness amid the pandemic. Many were cut off from affirming spaces, especially those who did not have a supportive home environment or had to hide their gender diverse identity. Some faced domestic violence and trauma at home yet had no escape. In addition to not having their psychological needs met, LGBTQ+ face a great deal of stigma, often from families, in school, and from the local community. Consequently, they also have a higher risk of depression, anxiety, suicide, and substance abuse, with the highest risk faced by trans youth. This is due to outright discrimination, victimization, and rejection. In response, LGBTQ+ youth often engage in negative coping strategies including substance abuse and self-harm.

Miller (2025) provides a concise overview of the minority stress model as applied to the mental health of sexual and gender minorities. In addition to experiencing prejudice and discrimination, LGBTQ+ also internalize the stigma of homophobia and will often feel the need to conceal their identity. All of these factors are associated with poor mental health. In addition, LGBTQ+ young people often have few social supports, especially among family members, educators, and even spiritual or religious leaders. The degree of neighborhood cohesion (or community solidarity) is also important to understanding the stigma and social supports available to LGBTQ+ (see Box 8.1).

BOX 8.1 Latina LGBTQ+ Youth

Schmitz et al. (2020) provide an account of the experience of Latina LGBTQ+ youth and develop the framework for an intersectional minority stress framework. In-depth interviews with 40 young people (aged 18–26) living in the Rio Grande Valley (a largely rural border community) demonstrate the effects of interlocking sources of marginalization and stigma (gender, ethnicity, immigration, sexuality) on their mental health. Everyone struggled to develop a strong sense of self-identity and resilience in face of a variety of mental health challenges. Of interest was the role of Latina familial and cultural traditions, which often intersected with religious values to increase the stigma of a LGBTQ+ identity. Some young people consequently rejected the church, though many held onto their religious values, finding resilience in prayer and spirituality. The study is rich in description and allows the voices of young people negotiating complex sources of stigma to be heard. The researchers point to the psychological toll of the daily effort to affirm intersectional marginalized identities, as described in the quotes from two young people they interviewed (p. 172).

To be proudly a Latino and an LGBTQ person ... it makes it hard to identify as both because you are bringing some sort of shame to your community.

Before I accepted myself, I felt really bad and did unhealthy things to myself like not eat at all because I felt very depressed and I was in a constant state of anxiety.

Gender diversity, or fluidity, is increasingly common among young people but an unstable or ambiguous self-concept does undermine psychological well-being. Further, in a heteronormative context (heterosexuality the norm), assuming a nonbinary or gender fluid identity can lead to stigma and marginalization. In a longitudinal study of young women (aged 18–27) in Australia, a site more supportive of sexual diversity, researchers (Cambell et al., 2022) found that about one-third had changed their sexual identity at least once in four years. Psychological distress was due to adopting a stigmatized identity, while plurisexuality and biphobia constituted an additional source of stigma beyond homophobia.

LGBTQ+ youth also lack more general social supports, especially if they are not receiving affirmation of their gender diverse identity. Positive supports come from gender-affirming spaces, which often involved online support groups for LGBTQ+ youth given the social isolation of COVID. Researchers utilized QChat and found that online synchronous text-based platforms provided LGBTQ+ youth safe places to access meaningful social supports (Fish et al., 2020). Given the limited content of most sex education courses, marginalized adolescents turn to online spaces to seek information about sensitive issues regarding sexuality. Online communities can provide protection from homophobia, transphobia, and other barriers faced in their in-person lives. In this way, online spaces can become safe havens for LGBTQ+ adolescents to explore and ask questions about their sexual and gender identities without fear of stigma or embarrassment (Hillier et al., 2012).

Telehealth was another beneficial impact of COVID for LGBTQ+ youth. Online therapy made it easier to access not only psychological supports but also gender-affirming services. Telehealth has helped provide increased access to both mental and physical health care, though many issues remain as to its ability to reduce health disparities (Ormiston and Williams, 2021). Online support groups may be especially important for LGBTQ+ individuals who are from racial or ethnic minorities. Black and Hispanic communities have stronger cultural norms that affirm traditional male and female gender roles, and so youth of color who are LGBTQ+ experience multiple sources of stigma and marginalization. These young people must engage in intensive emotional labor to navigate familial prejudice and microaggressions from teachers and schoolmates, and from their churches (Schmitz et al., 2020). Online chat rooms may be the only safe place to find a sense of community. However, online chat rooms or telehealth will not meet all the needs of minority and marginalized youth. Physical and mental health services need to be integrated so that assessments of mental health do not require a visit to a specialty clinic or provider. School-based services are also critical. Health providers, counselors, and teachers all need to be educated about not only the specific mental health concerns BIPOC and LGBTQ+ youth face, but about intersectionality and an understanding of identity development, diversity, inclusion, and equity. Young women and BIPOC individuals who are grappling with their sexual identity will need additional mental health supports in the face of considerable stigma as well as uncertainty. The lack of mental health supports is a major hurdle, as documented by the Youth Action Research Group, operating out of Montreal, Quebec Canada (Nichols and Malenfant, 2022).

The Youth Action Research Group (YARR) is an excellent example of participatory action research, where those who are affected by a given social problem (in this case youth homelessness) work with researchers to collect data as well as to develop policy initiatives to help solve the problem. YARR consisted of one professor, one graduate student who had experienced homelessness, and a team of four youth researchers who interviewed 38 homeless youth (aged 16–29) between 2018 and 2021. The interviews were extensive and sought to understand the intersection of mental health and homelessness. The young people they interviewed had histories of childhood abuse and trauma, compounded by traumatic experiences living on the streets. Unhoused youth not only had higher rates of MHPs and substance abuse, but also poorer physical health and high rates of sexually transmitted diseases. They faced multiple barriers to both mental and physical health care, which is surprising given Canada's universal health care system. However, health care services failed to provide any social supports or integration into the community, releasing a young person from a hospital to the streets. Services were also delivered according to a binary division, so young people who were trans or gender fluid faced significant barriers and outright stigma and discrimination. The authors (p. 152) concluded that the

> "failure to access high quality and effective mental health and addictions treatment can cause a person's homelessness... Furthermore, a failure to include access to safe and appropriate housing as an integral component of successful health interventions for young people undermines what might otherwise be an effective treatment option."

The lack of housing created another source of "othering" interacting with poverty, trauma, poor mental and physical health, substance use, and biphobia. The recommendations for solutions were to provide housing as well as accessible outpatient mental health services. In addition to prioritizing youth autonomy and choice, peer navigators and social workers trained in crisis intervention and de-escalation can have a positive effect and reduce episodes of confrontation and conflict arising from mental health or substance abuse problems.

Concluding Thoughts

The past decades have brought increased attention to racial and gender diversity, with fluid lines between what have been socially constructed rigid boundaries. Social change always involves conflict between what was once considered "normal" and the new "normal." Once referred to as identity politics, current efforts to promote diversity, equity, and inclusion involve fundamental changes to ways of thinking as well as social structures. There is notable pushback, as vested interests seek to maintain the status quo. One of Dr. Scheid's favorite quotes is paraphrased from Clifford Geertz, a noted anthropologist: people "pack the dykes of their most cherished beliefs with whatever mud they can find." In the United States, we live in a conservative political environment with school boards banning books about racial inequality and gender diversity, including books widely held to be classic such as Tony Morrison's *Bluest Eye*. Legislation has restricted access to gender-affirming care as well as prohibiting trans children from participating in sports based on their preferred gender identity. As of May 2023, over 520 anti-LBTQ+ legislative bills had been proposed across the United States (Miller, 2025). These legislative initiatives all point to the significant stigma of marginalized social identities.

Globally, we face the challenges of migration and immigration and also recognition of the salience of intergenerational trauma. These political conflicts involve intersecting systems of power, which also draws attention to the structural sources of poor mental health and distress. The power of socially devalued labels is another axis of stratification and intersectionality. Labeling theory and stigma are important explanations for the relationship between SES, minority status, and mental health. In Chapter 9, we turn to an extended discussion of stigma.

Student Activities

1. Review the Mental Health America's resources for BIPOC (a new toolkit was developed in July 2023) and those for LGBTQ+ youth. Provide a review and assessment of the information provided as well as how it was delivered.

2. Students could examine campus initiatives for diversity, equity, and inclusion. To what degree do these programs involve diverse voices in the development of campus policies? What can young people do to resist the stigma surrounding racial or gender diversity?

3. Explore the website for the Center for Intersectional Justice (CIJ) (www.intersectionaljustice.org). The CIJ is an independent non-profit organization established in Germany in 2017 with a focus on intersectionality in Europe. The goal of the CIJ is to reduce discrimination and inequality by linking research and policy initiatives with publications that provide data on intersectional discrimination. Of interest is that while the staff of the CIJ is small (less than 10), they post available jobs and internships. What things did you learn in your exploration?

References

Bowleg, L. (2012). The problem with the phrase: Women and minorities: Intersectionality – an important theoretical framework for public health. *American Journal of Public Health*. 112 (7): 1267–1273.

Campbell, A., Perales, F., Hughes, T.L. et al. (2022). Sexual fluidity and psychological distress: What happens when young women's sexual identities change? *Journal of Health and Social Behavior*. 53 (4): 577–593.

Fish, J.N., McInroy, L.B., Paceley, M.S. et al. (2020). I'm kinda stuck at home with unsupportive parents now: LBGTQ youths' experiences with COVID-19 and the importance of online support. *Journal of Adolescent Health*. 67 (3): 450–452.

Goodkind, J.R., Gorman, B., Hess, J.M. et al. (2015). Reconsidering cultural competent approaches to American Indian healing and well-being. *Qualitative Health Research*. 25 (4): 486–499.

Hillier, L., Mitchell, K.J. and Ybarram, M.L. (2012). The internet as a safety net: Findings from a series of online focus groups with LGB and non-LGB young people in the United States. *Journal of LGBT Youth*. 9 (3): 225–246.

Keith, V. and Brown, D. (2017). African American women and well-being: The intersection of race, gender, and socioeconomic status. In: *A Handbook for the Sociology of Mental Health*, 3e (ed. T.L. Scheid and E.R. Wright), 304–321. Cambridge, UK: Cambridge University Press.

Miller, G. (2025). Sexual and gender minority mental health. *Mental Health and Society: Theories, Contests, and Systems (previously titled A Handbook for the Sociology of Mental Health*) (ed. T.L. Scheid and E.R. Wright), (forthcoming). Cambridge, UK: Cambridge University Press.

Na, L., Ling, Y., Yang, L. et al. (2022). Age disparities in mental health during the COVID-19 pandemic: The roles of resilience and coping. *Social Science & Medicine*. 305: 115–131.

Nichols, N and Malenfant, J. (2022). Health system access for precariously housed youth: A participatory youth research project. *Society and Mental Health*. 12 (2): 136–154.

Ormiston, C.K. and Williams, F. (2021). LGBTQ Youth mental health during covid-19: Unmet needs in public health and policy. *The Lancet*. 399 (10324): 501–503.

O'Rourke, M. (2022). *The Invisible Kingdom: Reimaging Chronic Illness*. New York: Riverhead Books.

Paradies, Y. (2016). Colonisation, racism, and indigenous health. *Journal of Population Research*. 33 (1): 83–96.

Schmitz, R.M., Robinos, B.A., Tabler, J. et al. (2020). LGBTQ+ Latina young people's interpretations of stigma and mental health: An intersectional minority stress perspective. *Society and Mental Health*. 10 (2): 163–179.

CHAPTER 9

Stigma as a Fundamental Cause

Stigma is pervasive among societies and political systems. As described by the WHO 2022 *Global Mental Health Report* (p. 67 or Section 3.4), "the stigma attached to mental health conditions is universal, pervading across cultures and contexts and countries everywhere." Institutional or structural stigma refers to the societal level conditions and institutional practices that reduce the opportunities and resources that contribute to the well-being of those with mental health problems (MHPs). Structural stigma is indicated by the lack of community supports and resources not only for treatment but also for prevention of mental health problems. While we typically think of stigma as a consequence of mental health problems, in fact, stigma contributes to the development and experience of mental health problems (Grinker, 2021).

Stigma reduces access to those resources needed to avoid mental health problems as well as to deal with the negative consequences of mental health problems. As such it is a fundamental cause (Link and Phelan, 2001) and interacts synergically with the other fundamental causes described in Chapter 8. Synergies produce effects of which each part is individually incapable – so the negative effects of racism, inequality, and mental health stigma are more than additive, as implied by theories of cumulative disadvantage, and they are multiplicative, as reflected in the concept of intersectionality. However, the concept of synergy is somewhat misleading as it implies a kind of energy. In fact, individuals facing mental health challenges within the context of inequality, racism, sexism, homophobia, biphobia, and stigma experience a downward pull, or negative synergy. Stigma results in marginalization, social isolation, and loss of social supports, and for many, homelessness. When faced with multiple sources of stigma, one's self-concept is seriously undermined and resulting in fatalism, worthlessness, and hopelessness. Stigma also contributes to policy inertia, discriminatory laws and policies, and the lack of support for resources to address MHPs. Stigma resistance is a relatively new addition to the literature and is a potential source of empowerment and social change.

Sociological Theories About Stigma and Labeling

Stigma is a process by which a person is marked by a label that sets them apart from others and links that person to undesirable characteristics. A label is a definition, and when applied to an individual, it defines what type of person they are. The label of "mentally ill" is a highly stigmatized attribute that is deeply discrediting. Those labeled as "mentally ill" are seen as dangerous, unreliable, unpredictable, abnormal, broken, or deranged. With the links to behavior, the stigma of "mental illness" involves assessment of one's moral character. Many people associate "mental illness" with emotional weakness, a lack of control, and even sin. Defining who is abnormal, insane, or mentally ill involves moral judgments, with many seeing those with mental illness as not quite human. The determination about what is normal and abnormal varies from culture to culture, with abnormal behavior being linked to violations of social norms and expectations. Consequently, "mental illness" is often associated with deviant behavior and in most societies the label of "mentally ill" is a highly degraded status.

Public stigma is the way the general public views mental illness and involves common stereotypes that can result in prejudice as well as discrimination, just as public stereotypes about race and gender result in prejudice and discrimination. The public stigma of mental illness has resulted in segregation – the removal of those diagnosed with mental illness to asylums. However, more generally, public stigma results in social avoidance. Self-stigma is the internalization of public stigma and results in a loss of self-esteem, demoralization, and avoidance of others. Self-stigma can increase psychiatric symptoms and contribute to increased stress as well as difficult relationships with others. Odireleng, a young man from Botswana, describes how stigma stifled his recovery (WHO 2022, p. 57). "For the longest time I was afraid of speaking about my battle with mental health because of the stigma attached to it. Even after diagnosis, I had a very difficult time and lower self-esteem."

A potentially positive effect of the label of mentally ill is the receipt of treatment or services. Individuals with more severe MHPs or symptoms are more likely to be in treatment. However, numerous studies have consistently found that treatment benefits eroded over time while the stigma of being a mental health recipient remains (Rosenfield, 1997; Marcussen and Ritter, 2016), with self-stigma leading to increased social marginalization (Link, 1987; Harkness et al., 2016). This line of research supports what sociologists refer to as modified labeling theory; it is not only the MHP itself, but the label of "mentally" ill which results in stigma and lower self-esteem (self-stigma) as well as social rejection and reduced social opportunities (public stigma).

Labeling occurs at various levels. Individuals may self-label themselves as having a problem and seek care voluntarily. Thoits (1985) argues that much of what constitutes "mental illness" is emotional deviance, with inappropriate affect (emotional display) evident in a majority of DSM disorders. Crying, sadness, restlessness, and anger are all common emotional responses, but when we cannot manage our emotional distress, we display what Thoits refers to as emotional deviance. This is when our emotional display is viewed by others as inappropriate, for example, when we cannot stop crying, or are "irrationally" angry and hostile. Over time we will eventually seek help or treatment to manage "deviant" feelings and actions, often due to the pressures of others in our social networks. However, the perceived stigma associated with mental illness results in delays in seeking help, which cause an exacerbation of the MHP, as well as social isolation and even involuntary commitment.

Social reaction theory is relevant to understanding how other people label someone as having a MHP and in need of treatment. Social factors play an important role in who is labeled as well as who labels. Social integration, class, gender, race, and age all shape social reactions (Box 9.1). Individuals who are marginal, or have fewer ties, or who do not fit prevailing views of who is a "normal" person are more likely to be labeled. The greater the cultural distance between the labeler and the labeled also plays an important role, as well as the degree of marginalization of the one who is labeled. This is why the addition of stigma to other key social status characteristics that influence health is so important.

BOX 9.1 Youth Culture Viewed as Deviant

In an interesting study published in 1991 (Rosenbaum and Prinkey, *Crime and Delinquency*), researchers examined the effect of the cultural distance between adult and youth culture. They constructed a hypothetical situation where parents were concerned about their child's choice of music, clothes, and posters. A male research assistant posing as the youth's father called six public and six private inpatient psychiatric facilities over his concerns. No symptoms of mental illness were mentioned, and drugs, alcohol, depression, violence, and suicide were explicated ruled out by the "father." The majority of intake supervisors (83%) indicated they thought the youth's problems required psychiatric hospitalization, even though the only identified problem was involvement with a youth subculture. It does not take much imagination to understand how quickly a young person today displaying gender fluidity might be quickly taken in for inpatient psychiatric evaluation.

There is an increasing body of research on global stigma that shows an important link between cultural levels of stigma and individual stigma. The leading sociologist on global stigma, Bernice Pescosolido (2013: 15) has argued that "stigma is fundamentally a social phenomenon rooted in social relationships and shaped by the culture and structure of society." A biomedical view of mental illness is prevalent across the world and while viewing mental illnesses as having a genetic basis has led to increased public support for treatment (especially medications), those who believe mental health problems having a biological basis report higher levels of stigma. It appears that being biologically different is another source of "othering," which may be reduced with greater acceptance of neurodiversity. Neurodiversity emphasizes that differences are universal variations, and that society creates the ideas that evaluate some differences as desirable and others as undesirable, leading to labeling and stigma. Ideas about gender fluidity are certainly changing very quickly and will not be stopped by legislative mandates. Advocates of neurodiversity argue that society needs to confirm to the diversity of humans, rather than individuals conforming to societal stereotypes.

Anderson and Harkness (2018) examined the multidimensional nature of stigmatized beliefs. They found that people held diverse beliefs about mental illness, with configurations of beliefs about mental illness as chemical imbalance, genetic abnormality, bad character, or a consequence of stress as reflected in the biopsychosocial model. Stigma was assessed by "desired social distance" (i.e. how likely are you to want to avoid interactions with individuals with mental health conditions). They found that the beliefs that were associated with stigma varied based on the type of mental problem. Stress was associated with depression and genetic factors with schizophrenia. A belief in a bad character did increase stigma, but only in accordance with other beliefs for a given condition. An underlying point is that our beliefs about mental illness arise from our social environments, and recognition of this can help lead efforts to reduce societal or cultural stigma.

There is a stigma trajectory (Link and Phelen, 2001) with labeling being the first stage. It is important to note that mental health symptoms do not by themselves trigger labeling. Many who do have mental health problems are not labeled, and many without MHPs are labeled. We only need to remind ourselves of slaves who sought to escape their masters and were labeled with drapetomania. Blacks are still more likely to be diagnosed with schizophrenia and confined. Likewise, women in the late 1800s were more likely to be diagnosed with "nervousness" and confined to their beds; today women are still more likely to receive a diagnosis of anxiety or depression and a prescription.

The second step of the stigma trajectory is stereotyping, with the association of a variety of negative attributes attached to the label. This is where intersectionality becomes important, with multiple sources of identity intermingling and creating a collage of negative attributes. The third stage is "othering" with a clear differentiation between "them" versus "us." Othering is the basis for the loss of status, and viewing the "them" as devalued, inferior, and too often, as less than human. Discrimination, exclusion, confinement, punishment, and various forms of social control (forced treatment) are then justified as necessary. The stigma trajectory emphasizes that stigma is a reflection of power differences. It takes power to stigmatize, and stigma is a form of oppression. Multiple sources of "othering" intersect to create the conditions for more extreme forms of discrimination and social exclusion, including homelessness and incarceration.

Homelessness

We can illustrate the role of intersectionality and the stigma trajectory by examining homelessness. Whether houseless, or precariously housed, the number of people living on the streets, or in inadequate or temporary shelter is a multidimensional social problem that has sadly increased following COVID-19. The Opioid Epidemic and the subsequent increase in drug overdose deaths have also contributed to increased homelessness. Economic dislocation and the lack of affordable housing options are clearly the central dynamics underlying the persistence of homelessness. Most of us are only one paycheck away from not being able to make our rent or mortgage payments. The structural sources of poverty and inequality certainly play a key role in homelessness. Rates of drug overdose deaths are increasing for black men, pointing again to the importance of intersecting sources of marginalization. However, we tend to blame the homeless person for their "fate" rationalizing that they must have done something wrong. In the US evictions, efforts to "clean the streets," to empty homeless camps, and to incarcerate people who are homeless under vagrancy laws or for minor survival crimes all provide evidence of a lack of empathy, compassion, and community responsibility. At the most extreme end of a stigmatized identity, many view those who are homeless as less than human.

Our understanding of the extent of homelessness is limited to what a given community is able to collect from its homeless population. In the United States, data from the Department of Housing and Urban Development provide some insights. In January 2023, 650 000 people experienced homelessness. The majority of people (60%) who are homeless are in a shelter, or a transition program, or in a vehicle, leaving 40% living on the street or in an abandoned building. Half of the homeless are located in major cities, often drawn to some provision of services and not needing transportation to find food. Those who are homeless are also quite visible in larger cities where they lie on park benches or against buildings. Less visible are children who are homeless; they are more likely to be in a shelter with their mothers or living with another relative. About a third of those who are homeless are under 25, and their visibility is increasing.

The factors underlying youth homelessness include a history of abuse, trauma, neglect, or rejection, commonly referred to as adverse childhood experiences. Many teens and young adults are also rebellious and may seek escape from an environment they find too restrictive. A young person may have lost a parent or care-giver to COVID-19 or to a drug overdose death. Young people facing issues related to sexual or gender identity may also have cause to escape their homes, and to be homeless. As illustrated in Box 9.2, many young people turn to their pets for emotional support and a sense of mattering.

BOX 9.2 Building Bridges on Four Paws

In 2018–19, researchers (Schmitz, Carisle, and Tabler, 2021) wanted to explore the experiences of homelessness, mental health, and pets among LGBTQ+ young adults (age 18–25). The research project "Building Bridges on Four Paws" conducted in-depth interviews with 17 LGBTQ+ young adults who were homeless in two cities in Oklahoma. Previous research had found that 23% of young people who were homeless had pets that provided emotional supports. Relationship with pets is especially important for LGBTQ+ people to help manage the stigma they experience. Schmitz et al. (2021) found that relationship with pets was indeed a critical source of emotional support, which also enhanced their self-image and providing stability. In-vivo quotes from the participants in their study provide the main themes:

"They know when you're hurting and they're there for you."

"At least in this creature's eyes, I'm doing the best I can."

"Having pets has always been a ground rod for me."

Having pets also provided many of the study participants "an opportunity to resist these derogatory messages through sense of responsibility and commitment to animal care" (p. 13).

With the crisis in youth MHPs, parents or other caregivers may simply not be able to cope with the anguish of the young person in their household. These mental health problems are evident to teachers in the primary school system as well as into college, where many students are also unhoused or face food insecurity. In September, 2021 (the first full academic year following COVID-19), North Carolina Public Schools faced an "influx of homeless students" as reported by Greg Childress for NC Policy Watch (September 24, 2021). The state moratorium against evictions had expired on July 1, and thousands of families became "unhoused." In March of 2020, North Carolina School districts identified 28 000 students who were homeless and in the fall the number of students inadequately housed had exploded, with one district reporting 230 new homeless students in addition to the 500 who they had identified in the spring. A school social worker in the district felt the number could double before the end of the academic year with evictions when the state moratorium against evictions expired in July. Despite the obvious need post COVID-19, North Carolina lawmakers in the summer of 2023 were debating whether to make school lunches free for all students, so those who did not have access to food at home would not have to face the stigma of asking for a free lunch. Stigma is evident in our inability to provide the basic needs for those who are the most vulnerable, young people and people with MHPs.

Homelessness has been linked to mental illness, with rising rates of homelessness in the 1970s and 80s associated with deinstitutionalization and large numbers of people who had been "housed" in mental institutions having no place to go. Community supports and services were never developed, and Not in My Backyard (NIMBY) protests reduced the availability of group homes or other forms of supported housing for individuals with serious MHPs. While deinstitutionalization played some role in increasing homelessness, most people on the streets were not former mental patients. Instead, homelessness is a significant source of MHPs. Living on the street, or precariously housed in one's car, or a tent, or even in a shelter all produce severe anxiety, with few resources by which to escape. It is difficult to identify how many of those who are homeless meet criteria for a psychiatric diagnosis, but generally about a third are estimated to have a serious MHPs. Often substance abuse is involved, leading to significant co-morbidities.

One of the most systematic sociological analyses of homeless and mental illness is provided by Schutt and Goldfinger (2011) who examined the role of independent living as opposed to group living in promoting more positive outcomes in the Boston McKinney Project. The book provides an analysis of the importance of community integration as well as understanding sources of empowerment and autonomy. Group homes can foster a sense of community and shared decision making, but residents generally preferred independent living. Of interest is the role that conflict over rules regarding substance use played in the group homes. Participants who had substance abuse problems were often divisive and other participants and staff felt that there was a need to limit access to alcohol or drugs. The book is theoretically and empirically rich, and exemplary in its use of a diverse array of research methods to study a complex social issue.

Excellent insight into the experience of homeless people with MHPs who live on the streets of San Franciso is provided by Robert Okin (2014). Okin was the Chief of Psychiatry at San Francisco General hospital and also a professor of clinical psychiatry at the University of California, San Francisco. He had always been interested in people with severe mental illness, and when he retired from the hospital, he spent two years talking to homeless people on the streets, documenting their stories, and taking photos of them with their permission. As a psychiatrist he initially wanted to talk to those with mental health disorder, "but in time it became clear to me that a very large number of people I met didn't fit neatly into formal diagnostic categories...but they were extremely troubled, were doing poorly in their lives by any standard" (p. 5). Their stories reflect the combined problems of genetic vulnerability, poverty, difficult childhoods with trauma and abuse, and the trauma of war faced by veterans, drug addiction, and social marginalization. Each chapter in the book has photo and a firsthand account; for example Mary describes how "I Used to Live in a Home. Now I live in a Cardboard Box" (p. 37).

Okin not only provides important insights into the lives of the homeless mentally troubled, he points to the need for us to "be able to perceive the ways sin which we are the same, not just the ways that we are different. We'd be able to see that we all get cold when the temperature drops, that we all screw up and do things that make bad situations worse, take the wrong path, or fall off the horse and have trouble getting back on. And if we understood all this, we might feel more connected to the people we shun" (pp. 203–4).

A universal human priority is shelter, food, water and accessible facilities for meeting basic human needs. However, barriers to funding resources to provide these basic human needs have persisted for decades as the number of those who are homeless continues to grow. In addition, a major obstacle faced by those who are homeless and experience MHPs is the lack of community supports and mental health services. However, resources for meeting even basic human needs are limited, and often assistance to those who are homeless is provided by volunteers and non-profit agencies. In New York City ("The Street Teams in NYC which help the homeless mentally ill." NY Times, May 7 2023) street teams consisting of a psychiatrist or nurse practitioner, two peer support specialists, and three social workers provide a wide range of services to 27 clients. However, volunteers are often prohibited from providing needed supports.

Stephanie Southworth Brown, a sociology professor, began as a volunteer in Wilmington, North Carolina and she documented the many barriers she and other advocates faced in trying to provide needed services to the homeless, including a bike share program, providing sleeping bags, access to food and restroom facilities. She and her colleague Sara Bralleir involved their students in collecting data as class projects and published a book in 2023 based on their experiences and with over 250 interviews (*Homelessness in the 21st Century: Living the Impossible Dream,* New York, Routledge Press). She also involved her students in advocacy and in the fall of 2023 began to display the results of a photo-voice project where students worked with people who were homeless to take pictures and then describe their experiences. The hope is that students will go on to make needed changes in their own communities.

A major issue is the criminalization of homelessness, where individuals are not allowed to sleep in parks, or in tents, or even unauthorized trailers. If violating these rules those who are unhoused can be fined and arrested, adding to their inability to find stable housing or work. In Charlotte, NC, there has been continued debate in the City Council over how to deal with public urination in a neighborhood near where the library that had provided a public restroom was under reconstruction. Private property rights compete with a community response to homelessness, illustrating the division over competing values and priorities.

Stigma Resistance

Stigma exists at all levels – within the individual, in the reactions of those around the individual, in widely held views or public stigma, and in the social institutions within which we all live and work. Stigma is a significant barrier to community integration, housing, and employment and efforts to reduce stigma will go a long way toward promoting the goals of recovery. However, numerous efforts to address stigma, both in the United Kingdom and the United States, have not been very successful (Green, 2009). An important sociological idea is that of stigma resistance. Thoits and Link (2016) thought that stigma resistance could be an important coping strategy that might enhance well-being for those living with serious mental health conditions. Their research provides an elaboration of the stress process model, where stressors can activate coping mechanisms, which then mediate the negative consequences of stress on mental health. Stigma-related stressors include public devaluation, discrimination, and internalized stigma. The mental health outcome of well-being included subjective well-being (an emotional responses including happiness); psychological well-being (self-esteem, control, purpose, and autonomy); the absence of depression; and overall quality of life.

Three different strategies to cope with stigma-related stressors were studied. The first is simply concealing one's MHPs via secrecy or avoiding contact with others. The other two are both stigma resisting strategies, either challenging or deflecting stigma. Challenging occurs when individuals show they can perform social roles, educating others, or confronting biases. Deflecting is ascertaining that common public conceptions/stereotypes do not apply to them, such as "I am not dangerous." Both stigma resistance strategies pose some risk of increasing the likelihood of negative reactions from others who will respond to the label and not the actual behavior.

The data were from the Stigma and Psychosis Study, which interviewed 65 patients from three psychiatric hospitals (two in NYC, one in New Jersey). All of the patients were diagnosed with schizophrenia, schizo-affective disorder, or psychosis and had five or fewer hospitalizations. Thoits and Link (2016) found that stigma resistance did lead to higher levels of well-being, with deflecting having stronger effects than challenging. Those who felt they were no longer "mentally ill" (even though hospitalized at the time of the interview) had the highest levels of well-being. Patients who "hid" their mental illnesses had poorer self-esteem and depression, and these two outcomes were related.

A major issue is the degree to which people's sense of identity incorporates stigmatized social labels (internalized stigma), leading to social avoidance and concealment. The broader issue is that stigma resistance can be seen as both cause and consequence of rejecting stigmatized social labels. Drawing on Goffman's ideas about mental illness as a "spoiled identity" and identity theory, Marcussen, Gallagher, and Ritter (2019) focus on the relationship between "self-views" (how we view ourselves) and the appraisals of others (how we perceive others view us). Do you see yourself in terms of your mental illness as opposed to reflected appraisals where others see you in terms of your mental illness? They conducted in-depth interviews with adults in outpatient community mental health care and found that while self-views and stigmatized appraisals are positively associated, they have different mental health outcomes. Self-stigma results in lower self-esteem and efficacy, while the perception of stigma from others (reflected appraisals) results in higher levels of depression.

Given that those who accepted the label of "mentally ill" (i.e. my mental illness is a major part of who I am) had poorer self-evaluation and greater distress, the researchers argue that stigma resistance may in fact be a source of self-esteem. They explore this issue in a more recent paper where they examine the role of identity as mediating the relationship between stigma and well-being (Marcussen, Gallagher and Ritter, 2021). In this paper, the researchers develop ideas related to identity discrepancy, which is when your self-view is not verified by the social view, or how others view you. They then examine the role of identity discrepancy in the use of resistance strategies. Stigma resistance may be a way to reduce the discrepancy between one's view of themselves (I am not dangerous) and the views others have of you (I think you are potentially dangerous). What is interesting in their data is that 50% of their respondents had a more positive self-view, while 42% had a more negative self-view and only 8% reported no discrepancy between their views of themselves and the appraisals of others. They did find stigma resistance to be positively associated with well-being, and that "challenging stigma through activism showed promise in our study" (p. 31).

An important distinction between their study and the earlier study by Thoits and Link is that Marcussen et al. interviewed patients in community-based care, as opposed to hospitalized patients in the Thoits/Link study. Often community-based care can provide pathways to advocacy (i.e. challenging strategies) with bridging links to organizations such as NAMI or MHA (as we discussed in Chapter 5 from our book, *Ties That Enable*). Hospitalized patients have less control over decisions and fewer opportunities for stigma resistance.

Developing coping strategies to deal with stigma is also an important role for mental health providers and peer supports. Dobransky (2019) describes the activities of mental health providers as they work with clients to manage the stigma of mental illness. Based on in-depth interviews, he finds mental health providers engage in two strategies to help their clients.

1. Brokering/buffering: They protect clients from negative social reactions, which involve avoidance or withdrawal and providing more inclusive social supports (i.e. within the mental health care system, such as clubhouses) or consumer run groups. These strategies were more often used by providers working with clients with serious MHPs.

2. Normalization: A client-centered approach where clients are advised to share their problems with discretion. These strategies were most often used by primary care providers, who worked with clients with less serious mental health issues.

Dobransky found that providers helped their clients to both "normalize" stigma by helping them decide when (and who) to disclose their status to, and to "buffer" their clients from the negative reactions of others. At the same time, he found very little evidence of challenging stereotypes or activism among mental health providers.

Peer support groups and advocacy organizations also play an important role in promoting stigma resistance by challenging the common labels. Green (2009) reviews evidence as to the positive effects of peer support programs that lead to greater empowerment, and peer support programs are also identified as important to community integration by the 2022 World Mental Health Reports. Challenging strategies attempt to change the views of others and can be utilized as a primary form of advocacy by a wide variety of groups, including professionals, peer supports, schools, and churches. Resistance strategies can also provide a positive identity as well as improve prospects for socioeconomic status.

Stigma ultimately needs to be reduced at the societal or structural level. Grinker (2021) describes efforts in Japan to destigmatize schizophrenia. A non-profit established in 1984 to help people with schizophrenia (The Bethel House) hosts a yearly event, the "Hallucinations and Grand Delusions Grand Prix." This is a two-day community event designed to celebrate differences by giving people a space to express what they are thinking and feeling. The Grand Prize is given to the person whose "delusions or hallucinations contributed the most to the social cohesion and social supports of Bethel House" (p. 212). Such community-level stigma resistance is clearly linked to efforts in both the social disability and the neurodiversity movements to change the social structures, which view those with mental health problems as "less than" and which celebrates differences as positive.

Concluding Thoughts

Okin (2014) described the interaction between social stigma and self-stigma, where the people on the street he talked to internalized the negative labels associated with homelessness and mental illness. Sociologists have focused on the relationship between social and self-stigma and have addressed various strategies to resist stigma, including avoidance, concealment, and resistance. Avoidance of those who are different only reinforces stigma and also reduces potential forms of social support. Concealment also reinforces self-stigma and results in lower overall well-being. As Grinker (2021: 320) argued that while stigma is impossible to end, "we must still resist, name, mute, and shape it. Stigma is not a thing, but a process, and we can change its course." Stigma resistance shows promise as there is an acceptance of one's identity and also a focus on affirming a positive sense of self and accomplishment, which leads to overall well-being. Stigma resistance and its relationship to one's sense of self (identity) have important implications for understanding the experience of marginalized individuals and groups and also points to directions for positive social change via advocacy. Reducing stigma involves more than compassion; it is seeing others as worthy of the same things you enjoy without thinking about it. It involves humanization, caring, and recognition of the need to provide for inclusive places for everyone.

Student Activities

1. Students should explore depictions of mental illness (and/or homelessness) in recent movies and television shows. To what degree are processes of labeling, stigma, and stigma resistance evident?

2. Students should discuss their agencies in their own community that are involved in stigma resistance campaigns. In the United States, Mental Health America and the National Alliance of Mental Illness both have state and local chapters that are involved in efforts to reduce stigma. In the United Kingdom, the Mental Health Alliance (a coalition of 75 advocacy groups) works to reduce discrimination and advocate for the civil rights of people with mental health problems.

3. In the spring of 2024, the US Supreme Court heard a case (originating in Portland, Oregan) to determine whether criminalizing homelessness (i.e. laws against sleeping or camping outside) violate the 8th Amendment of the US Constitution, which prohibits cruel and unusual punishment. The case was decided in May, and the Supreme Court ruled that cities could remove people who were sleeping outdoors even if they had no other place to go. Students should examine the case and reactions to it, as well as the rules and punishments for those who are unhoused in their own communities.

References

Anderson, M. and Harkness, S. K. (2018). When do biological attributions of mental illness reduce stigma? *Society and Mental Health*. 8 (3): 175–194.

Dobransky, K. (2019). Breaking down walls, building bridges: Professional stigma management in mental health care. *Society and Mental Health*. 9 (2): 228–242.

Green, G. (2009). *The End of Stigma? Changes in the Social Experience of Long-Term Illnesses*. New York, NY: Routledge.

Grinker, R. R. (2021). *Nobody's Normal: How Culture Created the Stigma of Mental Illness*. New York: WW Norton.

Harkness, S. K., Krosta, A. and Pescosolido, B. (2016). The self-stigma of psychiatric patients: implications for identities, emotions, and the life course. In *50 Years After Deinstitutionalization: Mental Illness in Contemporary Communities. Advances in Medical Sociology*, (ed. B. L. Perry). 17: 207–334. Bingley, UK: Emerald Group Publishing Limited.

Link, B. G. (1987). Understanding labeling effects in the area of mental disorder: An assessment of the effects of expectations of rejection. *American Sociological Review.* 52: 96–112.

Link, B. G. and Phelan, J. C. (2001). Conceptualizing Stigma. *Annual Review of Sociology.* 27 (1): 363–85.

Marcussen, K. M. and Ritter, C. (2016). Revisiting the Relationships Among Community Mental Health Services and Well-Being. In *50 Years After Deinstitutionalization: Mental Illness in Contemporary Communities.* Howard House, (ed. B. L. Perry). 177–2016. UK: Emerald.

Marcussen, K., Gallagher, M. and Ritter, C. (2019). Mental illness as stigmatized identity. *Society and Mental Health.* 9 (2): 211–227.

Marcussen, K., Gallagher, M. and Ritter, C. (2021). Stigma resistance and well-being in the context of mental illness identity *Journal of Health and Social Behavior.* 62 (1): 19–36.

Nicols, N and Malenfant, J. (2022). Health system access for precariously housed youth: A participatory you research project. *Society and Mental Health.* 12 (2): 136–154.

Okin, R. (2014). *Silent Voices: People with Mental Disorders on the Streets.* Golden Pine Press, Mill Valley, CA.

Pescosolido, B. A. (2013). The public stigma of mental illness: What do we think; What do we know; What can we prove? *Journal of Health and Social Behavior.* 54 (1): 1–21.

Rosenbaum, J. L. and Prinsky, L. (1991). The presumptiion of infuence: Recent Responses To Popular Music Subcultures. *Crime and Delinquency.* 37 (1): 528–535.

Rosenfield, S. (1997). Labeling mental illness: The effects of received services and perceived stigma on life satisfaction. *American Sociological Review.* 62 (4): 660–672.

Schutt, R. K. and Goldfinger, S. M. (2011). *Homelessness, Housing, and Mental Illness.* Cambridge, MA: Harvard University Press.

Schmitz, R. M., Carlisle, Z. T. and Tabler, J. (2021). Companion, friend, and four-legged fur ball: The role of pets in the lives of lgbtq+ young people experiencing homelessnes. *Sexualities.* 1–23. doi: 1177/135346072098 86908.

Thoits, P. (1985). Self-labeling processes in mental Illness: The role of emotional deviance. *American Journal of Sociology.* 91 (2): 221–249.

Thoits, P. and Link, B. (2016). Stigma resistance and well-being among people in treatment for psychosis. *Society and Mental Health.* 6 (1): 1–20.

PART 4

The Complexities of Care

Mental health care is complex, with a variety of different types of patients, professional groups who provide care, and diverse systems of care. In addition, financing of mental health care is often confusing and inadequate. Finally, stigma serves as a major barrier to treatment and mental health care. Individuals may delay seeking care for fear of being labeled, families and communities are reluctant to acknowledge mental health problems, and societal level stigma reduces public support for programs that can provide mental health care and social supports. We examine the general framework of mental health care and treatment in Chapter 10.

As we noted in Chapter 1, people with mental health problems fall into three groups. The first group are those with acute (i.e. short-term) mental health problems such as normal depression following a loss or some other stressful event. Most of us will fall into this group at some time in our lives. The second group are those with acute mental health problems that are more severe, or those with chronic conditions who can maintain normal role functions most of the time. The third group are those with serious, chronic, or persistent mental health conditions that involve significant functional disability.

Treatment for the first and second groups primarily consists of medication and some therapy, with the second group seeking recovery with both a reduction of symptoms and a return to their daily activities and role functions. It is the third group, those with severe and chronic problems, that poses the major problem for mental health delivery systems, as they face significant functional limitations and need a broad array of services. In addition to needing formal mental health care for their mental health problems, they need a wide variety of social supports in order to deal with aspects of daily living. In Chapter 11, we examine the various forms of mental health care for those experiencing severe mental health problems.

Critical to mental health care is whether mental health treatment is voluntary or involuntary. Under what circumstances is coercion justified? What role should people with serious mental health problems play in making decisions about how to live their lives? Do they have a right to refuse treatment, including medications? Central to these questions is the social response to those with mental health problems, which leads us back to stigma and labeling. Rather than putting resources into community supports, we have been content to let the criminal justice system provide social control to keep troublesome individuals out of our communities, even though the costs of criminalization are much higher than those of community-based supports. In Chapter 12, we turn to some of the key debates over the use of coercion and social control.

Learning Resources

Students should view, or review, episodes from the PBS documentary *The Mysteries of Mental Illness: Explore the Evolution in Understanding Mental Illness*. A quick summary of the four episodes is provided in Appendix A. The series does an excellent job covering the history of mental health treatment and current issues and concerns that we address in the following chapters.

What things stood out to you in the historical accounts of our definitions and treatment of mental health problems?

What did you learn about the roles of social context and stigma in shaping mental health care?

CHAPTER 10

Mental Health Care and Treatment

Mental health care is provided by a number of different types of "providers" (people who provide mental health care) as well as in a diverse array of treatment settings. Mental health providers come from a wide variety of fields, including nursing, psychiatry, psychology, public health, and social work. Each of these disciplines has contributed to our understanding of what is needed to provide care, support, and treatment to those living with mental health problems (MHPs). Contrasting views of mental health treatment are organized around divergent views about the sources, or causes, of MHPs, which then results in disagreements about best way to "treat" these problems. Psychiatrists and nurses are likely to adhere to a biomedical model of MHPs and to prioritize medication compliance, while social workers and public health providers will tend to focus on the social environment. Psychologists are more likely to emphasize therapy and counseling. However, in practice, many mental health care providers adhere to an integrated biopsychosocial approach to care (Scheid, 2004).

Providing Mental Health Care and Treatment

Diagnostic psychiatry is based upon a view of mental illness as a discrete illness that resides in the internal physical makeup of the individual. MHPs are viewed as diseases or illnesses, reflecting internal dysfunctions or abnormalities. The source or cause (i.e. etiology) of mental illness is assumed to be biological, biochemical, and/or genetic (see Chapter 2). A clinical diagnosis meets defined clinical criteria such as those provided by the Diagnostic and Statistical manual (DSM). Individuals must exhibit certain symptoms for a specified period of time in order to meet the diagnostic criteria for any given diagnosis. Treatment consists primarily of medication (psychopharmacology) with less emphasis on therapy or psychosocial rehabilitation. Psychiatrists have a medical degree, and their primary role is to diagnose and prescribe medication. While all doctors are required to go through a clinical rotation in psychiatry, a psychiatrist is someone who underwent their advanced training in psychiatry. Damon Tweedy (2024:247) provided an excellent account of his training and background in psychiatry, and how he wished he had more training in psychotherapy. "All the years I'd spent studying microbiology, cell biology, and human anatomy seemed mostly useless when confronted with a crying patient." An excellent understanding of how psychiatrists and psychotherapists differ in not only their training, but understanding of MHPs is provided in T.M. Luhrmann's 2000 book *Of Two Minds: The Growing Disorder in Psychiatry*. Psychiatrists focus on medication, while psychiatrists who do psychotherapy undergo additional (and costly) training and a continued willingness to engage in their own psychoanalysis.

Many mental health providers take a middle road and emphasize an integrated biopsychosocial approach where medication is combined with therapy and basic social supports to deal with MHPs. Psychologists and social workers have contributed much to our understanding of recovery, building upon the view of MHPs as disabilities that can be overcome. Recovery is based on the goal of returning individuals to the community with models of psychosocial rehabilitation that work to develop basic social skills necessary for community integration. There is recognition that with effective medication, individuals with MHPs need more, not less, social support in order to maintain "normal" lives. Patients and advocacy groups also emphasize the positive role of both medications and social supports. However, there is also support for "forced" treatment to help individuals with MHPs whose actions and behaviors have become difficult to manage.

Sociologists view many mental health conditions as having their source in stressful life circumstances and point to considerable cultural and group variability in the experience of MHPs. Sociologists also argue that a reliance on diagnostic psychiatry and the DSM end up expanding mental illness to include many problems once considered normal, such as depression after a death or separation. Many MHPs are fairly normal responses to stressors and structural strains. The stress process model (see Chapter 4) posits that social context and status inequalities produce stress, which place individuals at greater risk for MHPs. Social status and race also influence diagnoses.

Sociologists also consider many MHPs to be a reflection of labeling processes. Social reaction, or labeling theory, asks two fundamental questions: who is labeled mentally ill, and what are the consequences of these labels? The label of "mentally ill" involves negative stereotypes and is highly stigmatized. Not only does the stigma of mental illness carry negative moral connotations, it can result in social isolation and withdrawal of the stigmatized individual and ultimately outright discrimination. Furthermore, because of the stigma of mental illness and the unwillingness of communities to accept those with mental illness, individuals are subjected to mechanisms of social control, coercion, and criminalization rather than treatment or therapy.

Legal scholars, sociologists, and criminologists have examined the criminalization of mental illness as well as issues related to coercion and commitment. Unfortunately, with the decline in community-based systems of care, the de facto system of care has become the criminal justice system, with far too many individuals with serious MHPs being warehoused in jails and prisons with minimal treatment. The central issue is how we finance mental health care, with far too few resources going to community care and prevention.

Paying for mental health care remains a formidable obstacle for most of us, from the worried well to those facing serious MHPs and functional limitations. Historically, in the United States, there have been two systems of mental health care: the private and the public. Private mental health care is funded either out of pocket or by insurance. Public mental health care is funded by federal, state, and local monies (generally via Medicaid or Social Security Disability) and supports services for those with chronic MHPs and groups who lack private health insurance. Beginning in the 1980s, private systems of mental health care became largely "managed" and public sector systems followed suit in the 1990s. Managed care emerged in response to rising health care costs and originated in the United States, but quickly spread to other industrialized countries. Managed care fundamentally refers to processes or techniques used by, or on behalf of, purchasers of health care that seek to control or influence the quality, accessibility, utilization, and costs of health care.

The result of managed care is that while mental health services have been offered by insurers, they generally had higher co-pays and deductibles and greater limits on services. In order to reduce this disparity in access to mental health care, the Mental Health Parity and Addiction Equity Act (passed in 2008) mandated that mental health benefits had to be offered on parity (on an equal basis) with physical health benefits. A major problem has been that insurers simply do not adhere to standards for parity and continue to work to deny or reduce payments for mental health care. These barriers became quite obvious in the wake of COVID-19 with the dual epidemics in MHPs and opioid addiction. The key problem is that the interests of insurers is to NOT pay for mental health care, either because of the desire to ensure profits (the private insurance industry) or because of scare resources in public sector programs.

While financing for mental health care in the United States has been extended with various mental health reforms, most notably the Affordable Care Act (2010), there are still many barriers to mental health care. Emphasis has been placed on the cost-savings associated with managed care and there has been less research on the quality of care received or the continuity of care received for more chronic conditions. A number of researchers and advocacy groups have found that the needs of chronic care clients are not being met by managed care arrangements. This makes sense as the driving force behind managed care and privatization has been to reduce costs. The only way to do this is by limiting access to treatment and utilization of more costly services while encouraging the use of less costly services. Consequently, short-term gains in functional status are prioritized rather than the longer term goals. What this means is that you likely will not be able to afford your mental health care, especially if you need long-term care.

Seeking Help for MHPs

There are many directions people and societies can turn to for mental health care. There is the "formal" mental health care system, which consists of both general health care providers as well as specialty health organizations including hospitals, outpatient clinics, primary care providers, and a diverse array of mental health specialists (for example music or art therapists). However, in much of the world, most people also utilize "informal" or "lay" mental health supports, which include family, friends, and a diverse array of self-help or social support groups, many of which exist online. There is also reliance on alternative mental health care, a segment that is growing in the United States along with the self-help movement. Finally, a good bit of mental health care is provided in other social services sectors: schools, social service agencies, jails and prisons, and long-term care facilities. Religious organizations often provide needed mental health support on both a formal and informal basis (Scheid and Smith, 2021). In this chapter, we limit our discussion to the formal system of mental health care.

Within this large and diverse "non-system" system of mental health care, there are numerous "pathways" by which people access formal mental health care, with a major distinction between voluntary versus involuntary decisions to seek help. MHPs are unique in that "patients" are often pressured to seek help and may even arrive at an emergency room in the back of a police car or ambulance. We will look more closely at involuntary treatment in Chapter 12 and will limit our discussion in this chapter to so-called "voluntary help seeking" behavior. We use quotes around "voluntary" as often times with decisions about mental health care our "choices" are constrained by the social context in which we live.

There are numerous barriers to seeking help for a MHP; the first being that there is a great deal of misunderstanding about what constitutes a MHP. Is not sleeping, eating too much or too little, restlessness, feeling tired all the time, anger, or feeling sad a MHP? When does a behavior become serious enough to warrant treatment? Unlike many symptoms of physical illness, individuals may deny, conceal, or seek to rationalize their feelings and behaviors. Families and friends do the same. Stigma and negative stereotypes contribute to reluctance to "label" a behavior as a MHP. Even when a behavior is viewed as troublesome, generally it has to be seen as problematic, unmanageable, or "out of control" before professional help is sought. Instead, informal supports are widely utilized at the initial onset of troubling symptoms. Several years may go by before individuals or those around them realize some kind of assistance is needed to deal with a problem. Suicide attempts are often the first signal that some form of help is needed, and hence the pathway to care is the emergency room.

While we can talk about voluntary help seeking, we are generally not referring to a rational "choice" a person makes to call the local mental health center. Instead, individuals are often pressured by those around them to seek treatment. Generally, it is not those closest to an individual (i.e. family or friends) but more distant social connections. For young people in school the teacher is often the one to recognize a MHP. For adults, it could be a co-worker or supervisor, or it could be police who witness erratic behavior. There are then multiple "doors" as well as pathways by which an individual engages in mental health care or treatment. It may be counseling at school, or through an employee assistance program. It may be finding a mental health therapist or entering a support group. It may be via the emergency room or through the courts. Both inpatient and outpatient care can be voluntary or involuntary.

An important sociological contribution is the Network Episode Model that sees social support systems as critical to the process of mental health treatment (Pescosolidio and Boyer, 2017). The Network Episode Model begins with the social context of the MHP (referred to as the episode), which includes the social position of the individual (age, gender, race/ethnicity, work status, education, SES) as well as their personal health background and specifics of the MHP (severity, visibility, and duration). These factors are then important for understanding the activation of a given support systems, decisions about treatment, and ultimately what is referred to as the "illness career." Acknowledgment of a problem constitutes a redefinition of one's self and can involve an acceptance of the role of a patient, one who needs assistance dealing with a MHP. The illness career then moves to some form of treatment, which involves deciding on a given type of treatment (and there are many options) as well as a specific setting, agency, or counselor. This process is much more complex in mental health than in physical health systems as choices are often constrained by geographic location, availability of mental health care, and the costs of care.

A very insightful account of the diversity in inpatient mental health care is provided by Norah Vincent in *Voluntary Madness: Lost and Found in the Mental Health Care System* (2008). Vincent immersed herself in the role of a voluntary patient seeking treatment for her depression. She (p. 6) described her depression as the "malaise of our age I was morose at an age when a lot of people were morose. I was spoiled. I thought life was supposed to make you happy." She came to see herself as one of the many who were over diagnosed and over medicated "We switched, jiggered, and recombined, looking for that perfect pickle" (p. 7). She spent time in three different inpatient institutions: a big city public hospital; a smaller, Catholic institution in the Midwest; and an alternative hospital with a focus on intensive psychotherapy. Following Goffman's (1961) analysis of total institutions, Vincent describes the differences in both the patients and the providers at each location and their interactions with each other, pointing to the significant differences between public and private hospitals in the United States.

The patients served at the large public hospital were poor, more likely to be minorities, and the $ 400.00 day daily cost of care was reimbursed by Medicaid. Vincent was viewed by her psychiatrist and social worker as a "set of chemicals" and while she did not take the antidepressant prescribed, she saw an adolescent patient turned into a "chemical waste dump." She felt the overuse of medication was to make life easier for the staff, who had few resources and were largely disconnected from their patients. The structure of the institution and its dependence on public funding limited the power and autonomy of both staff and patients.

The Catholic institution was rural and served mostly white middle class clients who had private insurance. Patients here had more rights and were treated with respect, and there was an emphasis on therapy as well as medications. The costs of care were much higher ($ 1,400.00 per day) and her insurance company ultimately refused to pay. Vincent then admitted herself to an alternative hospital, where all patients paid out of pocket (referred to as self-pay). A key component of the treatment approach here is that the mind and the body were seen as interconnected. Consequently, there was an emphasis on exercise to produce a "natural high" with the release of endorphins. Vincent also received intensive therapy based on a cognitive behavioral approach that views MHPs as negative thought patterns that can be "unlearned." Currently many therapists utilize a form of cognitive behavior theory. Dialectical behavioral therapy is a relatively new approach that focuses on identifying negative feelings and emotions. Mindfulness exercises are used to enhance the ability to deal with negative thoughts and to enhance well-being. Obviously, this kind of therapy requires time as well as money.

With privatization of mental health care, there are endless options for those who have the resources to pay for it. However, even if you have adequate financial resources for mental health treatment, it can be very difficult to find a mental health provider or accessible treatment setting. Many mental health professionals do not accept private health insurance, much less Medicaid, further exacerbating problems with access to mental health care. Access to psychiatrists is especially daunting. Tweedy (2024) described how his appointments were scheduled for months and the only way he could fit in a client in an emergency situation was to forego lunch. He also notes that psychiatrists "are the least likely to accept health insurance" (p. 252).

The Mental Health Workforce Crisis

Today, we are in the middle of a growing shortage of mental health care providers. In analyzing the mental health workforce fifteen years ago, Morris and Lezak (2010: 105) concluded that "at a time of growing demands to transform mental health systems by doing more and doing it better, there are not enough mental health professionals to do it, period, and the shortages are likely to get worse in the near term." The Department of Health and Human Services reported to Congress in 2013 that 77% of US counties have a severe shortage of mental health workers, with 55% of counties (all rural) having NO mental health professionals (Gordon 2018: 358). These shortages have increased dramatically in recent years with the loss of providers due to COVID, high rates of turnover, and fewer students entering medical fields. Rural areas, both in the United States and globally are much more likely to have shortages of all health providers, especially those who are trained to work with children and adolescents.

In recognition of the crisis in the mental health workforce, the Global Alliance for Behavioral Health and Social Justice issued a White Paper in June of 2022 (*Reconceptualizing the Mental Health Workforce: A Principle-based White Paper with Strategies for Operationalization*). The report summarizes research that documents increasing global demands for mental health care, critical workforce shortages, and increasing rates of burnout among providers. The White Paper advocates three important components to improving and expanding the mental health workforce. The first approach is to enhance the ability of community and primary health workers to provide mental health supports and services, with increased reliance on peer supports. Critical is not only licensing and credentialization but also reimbursement for mental health services provided by a diverse array of providers working in different types of treatment settings.

The second component is to strengthen the ability of individuals and families to provide for care, as well as for other community groups such as friends, teachers, or even religious organizations. Once again, peer supports are identified as a critical component of community based care. The final component is to enhance the workforce infrastructure, including use of new technologies, application of evidence based practices, and use of multidisciplinary teams. The White paper points to concrete policy efforts, including the Biden 2022 Plan on Mental Health, to provide support for their recommendations.

Underlying each of the specific recommendations is the recognition that the mental health workforce needs more than specialists with formal clinical training. It must incorporate nonspecialists (peer supports, school staff, human service workers) as well as community members (family, religious groups, and businesses). The re-conceptualized mental health workforce will further the goals of health promotion and literacy, prevention, remission, and recovery. The report goes on to detail specific goals for each component of mental health care with concrete objectives and principles, strategies for implementation, and examples.

A major component of the Global Alliance recommendations for the mental health workforce is the increased use of peers as members of supportive mental health teams. However, peers must be trained and credentialed in order for their services to be reimbursed. Mental Health America has been active in promoting peer support development and has offered a number of webinars to advance workforce development of peers. There is a National Association of Peer Supporters who are also promoting increased use of peers to address workforce problems. At the same time, while prosumers (a term used to refer to peer supporters) can help alleviate some of the burden of mental health providers, they also face similar bureaucratic constraints as well as burnout and stress due to emotional labor of providing care. Furthermore, peers themselves are disempowered and stigmatized by their lived experience with MHPs. Reimbursement is an important consideration as well; prosumers do not need to be exploited to provide a source of cheap labor.

Cross-training is one way for consumers, peers, advocates, volunteers, and providers to develop treatment protocols in a collaborative setting. Cross-training workshops and modules involve educators, providers, consumers, and volunteers in interactive trainings with objectives and outcomes determined in advance by collaborative teams who work to develop the curriculum offered in the training (Scheid, 2015). In addition to learning about the diverse perspectives of each group, cross-training can provide information on available community supports at both the formal and informal levels, as well as opportunities for advocacy and efforts to change the system of care. Cross-training can be easily incorporated into many community and education settings and would be very useful on college campuses seeking to expand upon peer-based social supports for mental health (see Chapter 5). An important component to any cross-training is developing cultural competencies.

Culturally Competent Mental Health Care

In the United States, those who access voluntary formal systems of care are more likely to be women, white, somewhat older, and from middle or upper class backgrounds. Their mental health providers are also likely to share a similar social position, with the majority of mental health counselors or therapists being white women. However, people with MHPs are increasingly diverse in terms of gender, race, age, and sexual identity. There are also gender, racial, and ethnic variations in diagnoses as we have pointed out in pervious chapters. Ethnic minorities are much less likely to seek care, in part due to a lack of access or resources, in part due to stigma, in part due to discrimination, and to the barriers of cultural differences in language, values, and beliefs. In an essay published in the New York Times (May 21 2023) titled "Therapy was not something Black Boys Did," Ismael Muhammad writes that

> "some people definitely need therapy, I realized, but did not seek it out, like my extended family, many of whom were haunted by drug addiction and the pain of gun violence. But seeking it out in the first place seemed to me, like a blemish, and admission of defeat."

There is clearly a need for culturally competent care, where providers share similar values and assumptions as well as social position. Provider level cultural competence increases not only the use of mental health services, it produces better outcomes. Given the increasing rates of suicide and drug overdose deaths among black youth, there is an urgent need for more male and black counselors, especially in schools where problems can be quickly identified. However, with the shortage of mental health providers, it will be difficult to simply hire more people of color and from diverse backgrounds. Resources need to be allocated to educational programs to increase the number of mental health providers in marginalized communities, especially in rural communities. Not only education, but competitive salaries and benefits are necessary. Counselors and therapists need to be aware of their own biases and positions of privilege and should engage in self-disclosure and reflection in continued training in cultural sensitivity or humility. Peer supports can certainly fill some of the gaps, as can cross-trainings and more effective use of volunteers. Schools can also introduce students to role models, people with their own lived experience, either as speakers or through readings and podcasts. Damon Tweedy is black psychiatrist who provides a firsthand account of his "miseducation" in psychiatry in a frank and open manner that will appeal to college students.

Culturally competent care extends beyond the counselor to the agency providing services to a given community. Services need to be tailored to include cultural beliefs that challenge Western assumptions. The Western bias is seen most clearly in the reliance on psychiatric medications or other medical interventions such as electric shock therapy. Community level interventions are also needed, with scarce resources being used to not only hire more minority providers and prosumers, but to fund social marketing of information and resources about MHPs in the communities most affected. Once again, peers can be trained and paid to serve as "lay" mental health advisors. Clinics can be coordinated with local businesses or market days. In the United States, reaching out to barbers and beauty shops has been found to be effective means to communicate health information to black men and women about the risks of HIV and mental health concerns.

Finally, communities can prioritize a social welfare model that addresses core problems of poverty, homelessness, unemployment and underemployment, violence, and crime, which all contribute to MHPs. Advocates and stakeholders need to collaborate to develop local solutions, which can build resilience to help people overcome their experience of powerlessness. Much of this work is simply bringing people together to identify core issues, develop strategies to solve the problems, and provide resources to do both. Mental Health America has hosted a number of town halls and webinars to help communities solve their mental health crisis (for example MHA Town Hall: Make Insurance Companies Pay for Mental Health, Youth Town Hall on Mental Health Parity, September 26, 2023). In July of 2024 with the rollout of an updated BIPOC toolkit, MHA held weekly discussions to enhance understanding of how to address the mental health needs of marginalized youth and in October they held a webinar on meeting the needs of youth in rural communities. These webinars include young people (consumers) as well as advocates and mental health care providers and promote empowerment.

Globally, MHPs reflect considerable cultural diversity (Grinker, 2019). Culture defines not only what is normal, but what a "mental" health problem is with many cultures rejecting the distinction between physical and mental health (or the mind-body dichotomy characteristic of Western Societies). Even with acceptance of common descriptions of a MHP (such as depression or schizophrenia) the symptoms display significant cultural variability. The illness career also varies considerably, with individuals doing much better in more traditional cultures where there is less stress, more social acceptance, and more opportunities for meaningful social roles.

Another important distinction is between more individualistic verse communal societies. In Western societies, especially the United States, individuals are seen as responsible for their problems. There is a greater reliance on formal mental health care and a neglect of needed social supports (for example housing). In more communal societies, families play a greater role and resources are often extended to families to provide informal care and social supports. There may also be a greater reliance on spiritual or alternative forms of care as well as family-based therapy.

An interesting example of how divergent cultural beliefs about MHPs can influence treatment comes from Ethan Water's (2010) description of Sri Lanka. Sri Lanka experienced a major tsunami in 2004, with widespread destruction and death. In anticipation of the experience of post-traumatic stress disorder (PTSD), American counselors and therapists went to Sri Lanka in order to provide mental health counseling. However, Sri Lankans had no symptoms of PTSD, which is a diagnosis developed with the experience of American men in combat situations. Sri Lankans had a very different understanding of stress than those of the US counselors, and strategies to deal with the devastation of the tsunami were based on collectivist values, not individual therapy. As a communal society, Sri Lankans responded to the trauma of the tsunami by working together to rebuild their social structures. However, the counselors kept educating Sri Lankans about PTSD, believing it to be a universal as opposed to a culturally relevant diagnosis. Culturally competent care involves prioritizing the voices of people and meeting them where they are and not presuming a shared understanding of a given experience. This is difficult for professionally trained mental health providers to do, and once again points to the important role of peers with lived experience of the trauma as well as the need for cultural sensitivity.

However, as described in the WHO 2022 *World Mental Health Report*, the tsunami led to major mental health reforms and a significant expansion of mental health services between 2004 and 2021. The number of inpatient and outpatient settings more than doubled, and child mental health clinics in general hospitals grew from 2 to 26. The number of mental health providers was also significantly expanded, in part due to enhancing resources for training and education. As quoted in the WHO report (2022: Figure 5.2): "every district in Sri Lanka has mental health services infrastructure, compared with a third before the tsunami." No doubt this infrastructure helped Sri Lanka deal with COVID-19 and is an example of the positive effects of globalization. While not adhering to individualistic assumptions about mental health treatment, Sri Lanka realized that community-based mental health services were necessary in the face of collective trauma.

Concluding Thoughts

The Western medical model has become dominant around the world, with a much greater reliance on medications. There is also an expansion of Western models of managed care, including privatization of formal treatment systems with an emphasis on evidence-based outcomes for reimbursement. There has also been growth in self-help groups and organizations as well as more advocacy for mental health reform. Finally, there has been a global emphasis on recovery. Another "globalization" trend is that of increased immigration, fueled by COVID-19 and its economic impact, political polarization, and exploitation, and the ravages of climate change on not only local economies but also people's lives. Mental health providers in all countries will need to develop culturally competent "tool kits" to deal with the diverse array of people migrating in and out of countries and who have experienced considerable trauma.

Class Activities

1. Review Episode IV of *The Mysteries of Mental Illness*, which describes a variety of new approaches to treatment of MHPs, including a renewed focus on ECT, deep brain stimulation, and the use of psychedelics. How accessible and affordable are these treatments?

2. Review Part IV of the PBS 2022 documentary *Hiding in Plain Sight* for a very good illustration of the need for mental health therapists who share the same cultural backgrounds as their clients. The young people in the documentary come from widely diverse backgrounds, with different family supports, and they describe their experiences of diverse forms of treatment. The mental health professionals interviewed also make a strong case for prioritizing the voices and experiences of young people.

3. Students should examine the degree requirements for the various people who provide mental health care: psychiatrists, psychologists, nurses, and social workers. Also examine the wide array of counseling programs available. What are some of the notable differences? Is there evidence of an integrated biopsychosocial model of mental health and distress?

References

Goffman, E. (1961). *Asylums.* New York: Doubleday/Anchor Books.
Gordan, S. (2018). *Wounds of War: How the VA Delivers Health, Healing and Hope to the Nation's Veterans.* Ithaca, NY: ILR Press, Cornell University.
Grinker, R.R. (2019). *Nobody's Normal: How Culture Created the Stigma of Mental Illness.* New York, NY: W.W. Norton.

Luhrmann, T.M. (2000). *Of Two Minds: The Growing Disorder in American Psychiatry*. New York, NY: Knopf.

Morris, R. and Lezak, A. (2010). Workforce. In: B.lubotsky levin, *Mental Health Services: A Public Health Perspective*, 3e (eds. K.D. Hennessy, and J. Petrila), 83–114. New York, NY: Oxford University Press.

Pescosolido, B.A. and Boyer, C.A. (2017). The context and dynamic social processes underlying mental health treatment. In: *A Handbook for the Study of Mental Health*, 3e (eds. T.L. Scheid and E.R. Wright), 409–430. Cambridge, UK: Cambridge University Press.

Scheid, T.L. (2004). *Tie a Know and Hang On: Providing Mental Health Care in A Turbulent Environment*. Hawthorn, NY: Aldine deGruyter.

Scheid, T.L. (2015). *Comprehensive Care for HIV/AIDS: Community-Based Strategies*. New York, NY: Routledge.

Scheid, T.L. and Smith, M.S. (2021). *Ties That Enable: Community Solidarity for People Living with Serous Mental Health Problems*. New Brunswick, NJ: Rutgers University Press.

Tweedy, D. (2024). *Facing the Unseen: The Struggle to Center Mental Health in Medicine*. New York, NY: St. Martin's Press.

Vincent, N. (2008). *Voluntary Madness: Lost and Found in the Mental Health Care System*. New York: Penguin Books.

Waters, E. (2010). *Crazy Like Us: The Globalization of the American Psyche*. New York, NY: The Free Press.

CHAPTER 11

Cycles of Mental Health Care

This chapter focuses on individuals diagnosed with serious, persistent or chronic mental health problems (MHPs), who we refer to simply as people with serious MHPs (PSMH). Other terms used through the decades of community care are patients (individuals in psychiatric hospitals), clients (referring to individuals in outpatient care), and consumers (a term popularized by the patients' right movement). Some who were critical of coerced psychiatric care (anti-psychiatrist) referred to PSMH as "survivors." As described by Pruchno (2022, p. 11) "serious mental illnesses have the potential to impair a person's emotions, thinking, social relationships, and ability to take care of basic needs." In addition to the long term nature of their illness, PSMH face functional limitations and often need assistance with income, housing, transportation, and social supports to be able to live in the community.

As societies developed and underwent the early stages of industrialization with migration to the cities, institutionalized systems of care replaced family and community systems of care for those with serious mental health problems. Institutions received widespread social criticism for their primarily social control functions as hospital censuses grew throughout the first half of the 1900s and housed far too many individuals to be able to provide therapy. Deinstitutionalization began in the 1950s with pressures to provide care in the community rather than in mental hospitals. However, funding for community-based care never met the demand, and very few state mental hospitals actually closed. The basic failure was the inability to develop integrated systems of community-based care which met the many needs of PSMH.

Evolving Systems of Care for Serious Mental Health Problems

One factor which influences the type of care a given society can provide to PSMH is the degree to which a given social group is communal as opposed to individualistic. Communal groups and societies have generally been more able to include individuals with severe mental illnesses and to provide needed social supports, whereas individualistic societies are more likely to exclude those with severe mental illnesses and to provide more coercive forms of social control (Horwitz, 1982). Communal systems of care include home-based care as well as care in therapeutic communities. With family-based care, such as in Colonial America, there was no real distinction between mental and physical illness; individuals were simply sick and could not support themselves. Families provide needed social supports including a place to live and assistance with daily activities. Sometimes this care can be merely custodial (with examples of PSMH being locking away in the attic), but generally families provide emotional supports and a sense of belonging. Historically, while many forms of communal care persist, in the United States, and in most industrialized countries care moved from the more informal care of families and small communities to more formal systems of care in institutional settings, as we saw with Sri Lanka in the last chapter.

There have been four major phases of formal mental health care for PSMH in the United States, each shaped by different societal values, political preferences, and economic priorities. First was the phase of institutionalized care, dominant from the 1800s until the mid 1900s, during which the primary locus of care was the mental hospital. Second was a period of deinstitutionalization, with the removal of patients from state hospitals to the community (roughly 1950s to the 1970s). The third phase, dominant in the 1980s and 1990s, was community-based care with an emphasis on integration of the diverse community services and supports needed for individuals with chronic MHPs to live in the community. Public mental health care involves both medical and social welfare systems that are influenced by programs and policies which provide funding for treatment, housing, education, employment, and a myriad of social support services.

With the advent of managed care and an emphasis on cost containment and efficacy in the late 1990s, mental health systems began to undergo a process of privatization with agencies contracting to provide services paid for by federal or state funds. Currently mental health services emphasize recovery, with a focus on living with one's MHPs, but with a reduction of symptoms and an enhanced quality of life. The COVID global mental health crisis increased the demand for mental health services, at the same time we are facing a global shortage of mental health care providers. While the time framework will vary, other countries have also experienced these major cycles of mental health care, with forms of institutionalized care still persisting in most places, including the United States.

Institutionalization and Deinstitutionalization

As societies developed and underwent the early stages of industrialization with migration to the cities, institutionalized systems of care were developed. MHPs were not viewed as diseases, but as undesirable behavior that could be changed. Treatment was provided by psychiatrists in inpatient hospitals, generally referred to as asylums. As total institutions, mental hospitals provided for all of the patient's needs, including housing, food, treatment, medical care, and social interaction. Such total institutions served primarily custodial functions, involving social control over patient's behavior rather than therapeutic care. One of the first sociological critiques of such institutions was Goffman's (1961) book *Asylums*. He analyzed the conflict between staff and patient perceptions of the asylum and described how patients needed to conform to medical definitions of their mental illness. We see the same general logic in contemporary discussions of "normality" where patients must first gain insight into their mental illness (i.e. accept that they are not normal) in order to move beyond the institution to life in the community. Acceptance of medical intervention and medications is central to such insight and recovery.

Mental institutions received widespread social criticism for their primarily social control functions as hospital censuses grew throughout the first half of the 1900s and housed far too many individuals to be able to provide therapy. Hospitals were depicted in both the academic and popular press as being largely warehouses for the poor and immigrant insane (see the classic movie: The Snake Pit). Begun in a period of economic growth and political liberalism (1950s), deinstitutionalization reflected a preference for community as opposed to institutional care for PSMH. Deinstitutionalization was promoted by three different groups: (1) fiscal conservatives who wished to save public monies, (2) civil libertarians concerned with patient liberty and rights, and (3) community health advocates. However, psychiatric medications provided the real mechanism for the transfer of care from the hospital to the community as chemical restraints replaced older physical strait jackets. Over 400,000 patients were released from the late 1950s to the early 1980s and communities struggled to meet the demands for affordable housing and many formerly institutionalized patients ended up homeless. While the number of patients residing in mental institutions declined significantly, the number of mental hospitals remained stable, and resources were never directed to necessary community supports to allow individuals to live outside the hospital.

The Community Mental Health Centers Act of 1963 ordered each state to designate catchment areas to serve between 75 000 and 200 000 PSMH, and community mental health centers (CMHCs) were generally organized along county lines. Funding to CMHCs went directly from the federal government via the NIMH to local control of the CMHC, bypassing the state which controlled financing for state mental hospitals. This led to direct conflict between state and local authorities, with states continuing to fund public mental hospitals even as the number of patients being treated in these hospitals decreased dramatically. State legislatures expected local communities to fund outpatient care; however, the funding never matched the demand for services. Instead state mental hospitals continued to exist with a large portion of mental health dollars being spent on state hospitals which continued to serve those patients who could not survive in the community. Some state hospitals diversified and began to provide a wider range of outpatient residential services. Dowdall (1996) described the diverse array of outpatient services offered by the

Buffalo State Mental Hospital following deinstitutionalization and shows how some state hospitals provided comprehensive treatment for PSMH, including outpatient care, day programs, skills training, and partial hospitalization. However, in most communities underfunded and understaffed CMHCs struggled to meet the needs of the thousands of patients who were discharged from the state hospitals into the community. The failure of deinstitutionalization was the inability to develop integrated systems of community-based care which met the many needs of those with chronic MHPs in the community

Community-based Care

Concurrent with deinstitutionalization was the demand for community-based care and integration. Community care requires that basic needs are met in order for integration into the community to be realized, and integration requires a nonstigmatized, accepting environment. Community mental health centers (as authorized by the Community Mental Health Centers Act of 1963) were supposed to develop the skills and competencies of PSMH so they could live in the community, provide social supports in the community, and help reduce societal levels of stigma. These are all very lofty goals and obviously require comprehensive programs housed in the community. However, funding for these programs never met even minimal demands for more services. Instead, CMHCs served primarily the needs of clients with more acute mental health disorders, referred to as the "worried well." Communities were (and still are) unable to provide care for PSMH, who need a variety of supports to live in the community. There is often resistance to group homes and clubhouses being placed in residential neighborhoods. Stigma has remained a formidable barrier to community acceptance and tolerance.

Researchers pointed to the revolving door of hospital admissions, with patients revolving in and out of the hospital as they could not find or access needed community supports. Many simply lived on the streets and were quickly readmitted to the hospital. There were also administrative and system level barriers to community care. Communication channels between the courts, the hospitals, and the CMHC were at best incomplete, at worst nonexistent. Referrals seemed to depend on informal connections between individuals who worked together across organizational boundaries rather than formal procedures. The CMHC generally had no knowledge of patients being released to their care, even in the cases of a court order for outpatient treatment. CMHCs were not opposed to providing care for PSMH; they simply had very limited means with which to deal with numerous problems faced by PSMH.

More fundamentally, reimbursement for even minimal levels of community care was inadequate. In the United States, funding for community care is a reflection of federal policy and was restricted after the Reagan era block granting of the Alcohol, Drug Abuse, and Mental Health funds as well as Social Services funding (the 1980 Omnibus Reconciliation Act). These block grants limited federal funds and states, and local communities were held responsible for funding CMHCs, which resulted in wide variability in support from one community to another. In addition, changes in federal policies affecting housing and welfare funding also had detrimental effects on PSMH, leading to reduced social supports and homelessness. Few would disagree that funding was (and still is) inadequate, leading to wide gaps in services. CMHCs simply had neither the resources nor the capacity to provide for even the most basic needs of PSMH, much less to achieve the lofty ideals of community integration. Instead, the focus shifted to managing the costs of care, rather than providing care.

Beginning in the 1990s, both private and public systems of mental health care moved to managed care systems, with a greater emphasis on managing costs rather than care. Rather than providing integrated community-based treatment, systems of mental health care focused on controlling access to care. Managed care emphasizes cost containment, performance assessment, and measurable outcomes, and subjects the treatment actions of health care providers to increased scrutiny and organizational control. Managed care uses a variety of means to limit the access to services and the utilization of more costly services while encouraging the use of less costly services, resulting in a reliance upon short-term therapy and psychiatric medications. One psychiatrist the first author interviewed in the early 1990s spoke about the challenges of managed care "our society has defined success in recent times by productivity and numbers – a bottom line mentality which is opposed to the therapeutic process and dehumanizes the clinician as well as the patient" (Scheid, 2004).

In describing how their work had changed since the advent of managed care (Scheid 2004), mental health providers complained about excessive paperwork and difficulties with the management information system (a computer system which contains client data). Consequently, they were less able to provide direct client care. Providers reported a twofold increase in time spent documenting care and felt that efficiency was hindered by having all services needing to be certified by the review panel rather than the treatment team. One comment from a nurse Scheid (2004) interviewed demonstrates the impact managed care had upon her ability to provide care to her clients.

> *"The paperwork has expanded at least fourfold, and is taking additional time from patient care. There is not time to build a relationship with a patient or his family, and trust is lost, the frustration level in providing care because of cumbersome preapproval procedures and denials of needed services has increased to a level where I will be glad to leave nursing."*

Mental health providers were frustrated that treatment decisions were being made on the basis of cost, rather than clinical need, and that volume was a higher priority than quality of care. Almost all of the providers described the negative effect of cost containment strategies on the quality of care, and the "devastating effect of shortened lengths of stay for chronically ill clients." The emphasis on cost was felt to directly interfere with client care, and clients were getting sick and sicker. In response to a question about the problems with managed care one male case manager said that

> *"fiscal issues are more important than client related ones, there is a lack of information to ground level clinicians regarding changes, there is staff burnout – look at the number of new hires in case management over the last year. Case managers and other professionals have to fight for services, our hard jobs are getting harder."*

We once again hear all types of health providers are experiencing high levels of burnout with the onset of the COVID mental health crisis and increased demands for care.

The Dilemma of Recovery

Perhaps not coincidentally, along with managed care came a focus on client-based recovery. While difficult to define, much less measure, there are two distinct views of recovery. First is the biomedical view that emphasizes the reduction of psychiatric symptoms and a "return" to a normal life, that is, fulfilling normative expectations and roles. Generally, this is accomplished by the "patient" taking their prescribed medication. The biomedical view of recovery is promoted by mental health providers who focus on diagnosis and adherence to a given medication regime as a necessary first step to recovery. A second view of recovery is promoted by the consumer/survivor movement which emphasizes self-determination, agency, and improved quality of life, which does not necessarily involve resuming normal social roles. The issue of empowerment is problematic, and the dual meanings of recovery help us understand the conflict between providers and their clients over the meaning of empowerment in the face of organizational constraints which link service provision to compliance with treatment directives. While mental health care providers were facing the organizational consequences of managed care, PSMH were facing the daily reality of living with these two contradictory meanings of recovery.

The apparent political consensus over recovery is noteworthy, given the many debates over treatment for MHPs. Federal level initiatives such as the 1999 Surgeon General's Report on Mental Health and the 2003 President's New Freedom Commission on Mental Health set recovery as a standard for mental health reform. Recovery has become an established principle in other countries as well, although the lack of a clear definition and guidelines for implementation remain formidable barriers to its realization in practice. The National Consensus Conference on Mental Health Recovery was convened in 2005 by the Center for Mental Health Services and involved over 100 consumers, advocates, providers, and researchers. They developed a definition of recovery and articulated ten principles of recovery which include such goals as: self-direction, individualized treatment, empowerment, peer support, respect, responsibility, and hope (Anthony and Ashcraft, 2010). It is not surprising that so many espouse recovery as a worthy aspiration; the issue is whether recovery can actually be fostered within our current nonsystem of mental health care, or in those communities where individuals with serious mental disabilities would like to reside.

Recovery builds on the ideals of consumer empowerment and is based on an advocacy model first introduced by Rose and Black (1985). While a focus on patient rights was certainly important to the original community care movement, empowerment pushed the idea of client autonomy to emphasize the individual's right to advocate for their own care and assume control over the direction of their own treatment. Some advocates of empowerment even rejected professional intervention, building upon critiques of both biomedical and psychosocial rehabilitation models which ultimately wanted clients to conform to professional definitions of mental health (Paulson, 1992). The concept of empowerment has evolved from independence from the system to choice within the system (McLean 2000, p. 837).

Recovery involves both a reduction in psychiatric symptoms as well as recovery within illness with clients determining their own quality of life. We can think of recovery as a form of well-being for those who experience more severe MHPs or functional disabilities. Recovery involves the psychosocial conditions for leading a fulfilling life (such as hope, connection, and empowerment) as well as the external conditions which allow individuals to lead a productive life, such as housing and income supports (Jacobson, 2004). Recovery can mean an expanded service model as once an individual's symptoms are stabilized, they will have an increased need for social supports and skills building program (Neugeboren, 1999). However, recovery can also mean reduced reliance (and cost savings) on service systems when defined as meeting certain limited functional goals. Recovery can thus be used as a yardstick for improved client outcomes with little commitment to creating the kind of therapeutic environments where recovery can be fostered and maintained. Consequently, there have been few guidelines on how to implement recovery in practice.

Myers (2015, p. 13), in her ethnography of recovery, argued that moral agency, or the "ability to be recognized as a good person" is the "overlooked driver of recovery." She details the path to recovery, with step one being "Take Your Medications." Medication adherence is an evidence based "best practice" and is considered the primary means to insight and rationality. However, most psychiatric medications have notable side effects as Estroff describes so well in her much earlier ethnography (1981) when she took Prolixin in order to understand the client's perspective. Estroff (1981) and Myers (2015) concurred in linking side effects to further stigmatization. For providers, noncompliance is a major problem, while for PSMH, side effects are a major problem. It is no wonder that so many consumers refer to themselves as "survivors" of the mental health system.

Models for recovery have been expanded in the past decades to provide clearer guidance for as to what enhanced quality of life means for PSMH. The CHIME-D conceptual framework includes six dimensions: (Stuart, Tansey, and Quayle, 2017).

C: Connectedness
H: Hope and optimism for the future
I: Identity and a positive perception of oneself and how others view you
M: Meaning in life
E: Empowerment
D: An addition to the original CHIME framework, which recognizes the additional difficulties of stigma and trauma which influence personal recovery.

It is clear that recovery essentially involves enhanced wellbeing, and the subjective experiences of those living with serious mental health problems. Medical recovery is not necessary for personal recovery, and CHIME-D can be broadly applied to a wide range of contexts with adequate training and use of interdisciplinary treatment teams which include peer supports. However, recovery remains an idealistic goal, with few concrete resources being allotted to provide the necessary supports for successful integration into communities for PSMH.

Concluding Thoughts

Once again, a cross-cultural comparison provides a critique of medical approaches to recovery. Waters (2010) studied families' experience with schizophrenia in Zanzibar. As a reminder, the symptoms of schizophrenia, delusions, and hallucinations, are found in all societies and cultures at around a one percent prevalence rate, supporting a biomedical disease model. However, the array of symptoms as well as the content of delusions and hallucinations exhibit cultural diversity. Further, the course and outcome (i.e. recovery) varies considerably with people identified as living with schizophrenia doing much better in less developed countries. This could be due to lower stress, higher levels of social support, or less reliance on psychiatric medication. Zanzibar, consistent with the globalization trends described in the previous chapter, began to adhere to a biomedical view of schizophrenia with a reliance on medications as opposed to more extensive family-based supports. However, this medicalization resulted in higher levels of stigma, a view of those with schizophrenia as dangerous, and exclusion from family and social networks, mirroring processes we see in the United States and other industrialized countries.

It may be that medications will always be necessary for many PSMH. At the same time, medications are not the sole means to mental health; there has to be social supports and meaningful relationships which produce a sense of belonging and flourishing. While medications may function as a bandage for a sprained ankle, you need to eventually get off the couch and walk, but you need someplace to walk to (Neugeboren, 1999). In most counties, PSMH remain isolated and alone with few supports in the community, while some have found ways to integrate families into recovery-based models and to provide informal as well as formal supports. Other models can provide a sense of community, such as the contemporary therapeutic communities of Italy, or Fountain House clubhouses (described in Chapter 5). We also described the Bethel House in Japan, where the contributions of those who live with schizophrenia were celebrated during a yearly festival. These communities have emphasized empowerment as well as recovery and serve as important models for advocates of patient's rights to self-determination.

Student Activities

1. Review Part III of *The Mysteries of Mental Illness: The Rise and Fall of the Asylum* (reviewed in Appendix A). Asylums became places where people were not only "out of mind, but also out of sight and forgotten." What role did racism play in the treatment of people with MHPs?

2. Mental hospitals still exist across the world. Many hospitals also maintain psychiatric wards, and individuals admitted to the emergency room will often be transferred to a specialized

psychiatric ward or hospital. What kind of specialized mental hospitals or wards exist in your community? Provide a little history or background on one facility.

3. Examine policies and programs for recovery in your community or country, or perhaps a country you would like to know more about. Look for information about day programs, clubhouses, peer advocacy, and governmental initiatives. In the United States, local and national chapters of Mental Health America and the National Alliance of Mental Illness can provide local and regional information.

References

Anthony, W.A. and Ashcraft, L. (2010). The recovery movement. In: *Mental Health Services: A Public Health Perspective*, 3e (eds. B.L. Levin, K.D. Hennessy and J. Petrila), 465–480. New York, NY: Oxford University Press.

Dowdall, G.W. (1996). *The Eclipse of the State Mental Hospital: Policy, Stigma, and Organization*. Albany, N.Y: State University of New York Press.

Estroff, S.E. (1981). *Making It Crazy: An Ethnography of Psychiatric Patients in an American Community*. Berkeley, CA: University of California Press.

Goffman, E. (1961). *Asylums: Essays on the Social Situation of Mental Patients*. New York: Doubleday Anchor Books.

Horwitz, A.V. (1982). *The Social Control of Mental Illness*. New York, NY: Academic Press.

Jacobson N. (2004). *In Recovery: The Making of Mental Health Policy*. Nashville, TN: Vanderbilt University Press.

McLean A.H. (2000). From ex-patient alternatives to consumer options: Consequences of consumerism for psychiatric consumers and the ex-patient movement. *International Journal of Health Services* 30 (4): 821–847.

Myers, N.L. (2015). *Recovery's Edge: An Ethnography of Mental Health Care and Moral Agency*. Nashville, TN: Vanderbilt University Press.

Neugeboren, J. (1999). *Transforming Madness: New Lives for People Living with Mental Illness*. Berkeley: University of California Press.

Paulson, R. (1992). Advocacy and empowerment: Mental health care in the community. *Community Mental Health Journal* 28: 70–71.

Pruchno, R. (2022). *Beyond Madness: The Pain and Possibilities of Serious Mental Illness*. Balitmore, Maryland: Johns Hopkins University Press.

Rose, S.P. and Black, B.L. (1985). *Advocacy and Empowerment: Mental Health Care in the Community*. Boston: Routledge and Kegan Paul.

Scheid, T.L. (2004). *Tie a Knot and Hang On: Delivering Mental HealthCare in a Turbulent Environment.* Hawthorne, NY: Aldine De Gruyter Press.

Stuart, S.R., Tansey, L., and Quayle, E. (2017). What we talk about when we talk about recovery: A systematic review and best-fit framework synthesis of qualitative literature. *Journal of Mental Health* 26 (3): 291–304.

Waters, E. (2010). *Crazy Like Us: The Globalization of the American Psyche.* New York: The Free Press.

CHAPTER 12

Dilemmas of Care

The dominant treatment for mental health problems (MHPs) is medication, consistent with the biomedical model which views these problems as illnesses. Often the comparison is made to diabetes, which requires daily medications and treatment to be able to live. Just as with insulin, psychiatric medications treat the symptoms of mental health problems, but they do not provide a cure. The reason is that we do not know what the cause of the MHP is. As articulated by a psychiatrist Carlat (2010, p. 6) "we know almost nothing definitive about the pathophysiology of mental illness." Instead, we work backward from a drug that is found to relieve symptoms to try to figure out why it works. This is the origin of the widely accepted "chemical imbalance" theory which posits drugs work to correct neurological imbalances in the brain, just as insulin corrects metabolic imbalances in the body. However, while insulin levels can be easily monitored to provide precise information on the metabolism of carbohydrates and sugars, we still cannot find a similar physical marker for most mental health conditions. In this chapter, we examine issues related to the widespread emphasis on the medical treatment of MHPs, referred to as medicalization, and debates over whether medication should be "forced" on individuals. This leads us to a discussion of involuntary treatment and commitment. We end the chapter with a discussion of the criminalization of MHPs and the reality that many PSMH spend years in the criminal justice system. The fact that the criminal justice system has become the primary provider of mental health care is a direct result of a lack of investment in mental health care services and community-based social supports.

Medicalization

Medicalization involves adopting a medical framework to understand a social problem as well as acceptance of medical intervention as the primary solution to the problem. A number of social issues relevant to mental health have been medicalized, including addiction, alcoholism, eating disorders, learning disabilities, obesity, pain, sexual and gender differences, and trauma. Mental health is one of the most prevalent areas of medicalization because social and cultural influences are critical to definitions of mental health as well as mental health problems. In addition, the identification of a MHP is based upon behaviors. The term behavior health refers to both MHPs and substance misuse.

Conrad (2007) is the sociologist who has led the way to our current understanding of medicalization, beginning with his analysis of attention deficit-hyperactivity disorder (ADHD). An important extension of medicalization is the recent addition of adult ADHD to the DSM, which is now more commonly diagnosed than ADHD in children and adolescents. There are many social factors to account for the growth in rates of ADHD. First is the rise of both single parent households and those with both parents working with less ability to spend time with their children. In terms of education, the number of students in classrooms grew larger while resources for teachers and assistant teachers were shrinking. School recesses and opportunities for physical activity were also reduced. Urban areas faced a shortage of parks and safe places for young children to play, as well as the loss of dedicated recreation areas where teens could expend their energy as well as socialize. Sugar consumption increased with sugary fruit drinks replacing milk for children, and soft drinks widely consumed by teens. Medicalization is obvious in that the primary treatment for ADHD and anxiety is medication, rather than addressing these various aspects of the social environment.

The COVID-19 pandemic resulted in an increased use of medication to treat mental health problems. Using data from the CDC, the *New York Times* reported on the increased use of psychiatric medication between 2019 and 2021 (Coronavirus Briefing, July 11, 2022). In 2021, 77 million prescriptions for ADHD drug were written, a 6 million increase over those written in 2020. The use of ADHD drugs by adults aged 20–44 increased by 16.7%. Overall, the use of prescription drugs for MHPs had increased from 15.8 to 25% of Americans.

There was an 8.7% increase in antidepressants, and a 17.3% increase in the use of anxiety medications by teenagers. Clearly, COVID-19 was a major source of stress and trauma, and restrictions on office visits to health care providers made it easier (and often necessary) to prescribe medications. The "drivers" of medicalization identified by Conrad (2007) include the medical profession, social movements and interest groups, and patients themselves. However, the pharmaceutical industry and the bio-medicalization of MHPs has been a consistent force behind the reliance on medications. The pharmaceutical industry is one of the most profitable in the world and they exert tremendous control over the research and standards by which drugs are approved, authorized, and reimbursed. They also aggressively market drugs to physicians as well as the public.

There has been tremendous expansion in the numbers of mental health disorders described in the DSM, from 106 diagnoses 1952 to 265 in 1980 (DSM-III) and 298 in the 2013 DSM-5 (this Table is in Chapter 3). This is referred to as diagnostic inflation. These medical categories define who and what is "normal." In an essay published in 1994, in the New England Journal of Medicine, Clifton Meador worried that "eventually every well person will be labeled sick." We are pretty close to that prediction now with many human differences transformed into pathologies. Another major concern with medicalization is that normal responses to the world around us are also viewed as evidence of a medical problem. Anxiety and depression are normal responses to the stress of the COVID, to climate change, or to increased violence. An inability to sit still is normal in a sedentary society where we passively consume information and entertainment. Problems concentrating are normal responses to educational and workforce technologies that are often boring and repetitive. An inability to focus is a normal response to the hours of screen time most of us engage in.

Psychiatric drugs do provide some relief of symptoms, and thus are viewed as a "magic bullet" by both patients and health providers. Thorazine certainly transformed mental health care, allowing for many patients to be moved from psychiatric hospitals to the community. Thorazine was developed as a muscle relaxant and was quickly reinvented as a mood stabilizer as patients were no longer acting out. Kolker (2020, p. 87) noted that "even today no-one knows for sure why Thorazine and other neuroleptic drugs do what they do." The dopamine hypothesis has been offered, arguing that the psychiatric drugs affect dopamine levels. However, Thorazine decreases dopamine and a newer drug, which is very successful with some patients, Clozapine, increases dopamine. While both drugs work for some patients, we have few insights into which patients will benefit from a given drug, or what the appropriate dosage might be, or how long a patient will need to take a medication. The psychiatrist often serves as an alchemist, trying one drug, then another and often adding different drugs to a cocktail to deal with a diverse array of symptoms and side effects. Tweedy (2024, p. 229) described a female patient with a history of assault he saw at a VA hospital who had been prescribed "a Noah's ark of psychiatric medications."

Whitaker (2010) reviewed 50 years of patient outcome data and found that patients actually did better *without* psychiatric medications. Even patients diagnosed with schizophrenia who were not medicated did better, with a higher recovery rate as measured by being able to live in the community. This may be one reason that individuals diagnosed with schizophrenia do better in less developed countries, where there is far less reliance on psychiatric drugs. Likewise, Whitaker (2010) argued that while benzodiazepines (used to treat anxiety and mood disorders) can provide short-term effects by "numbing" psychiatric distress, long term use can actually increase anxiety and depression as well as leading to cognitive impairment. This is termed an iatrogenic effect, where the medication (or any other treatment) can actually create new health problems. More troubling is that long-term use of psychiatric medications for bipolar disorder, depression, and schizophrenia has been linked to lower life expectancies of 10–15 years due to physical health problems, including heart disease. A further concern is that when many people are quickly administered psychiatric drugs, it is becoming impossible to actually examine the long term effects of medications as compared to control groups who have not received medication. We have no way to assess the long-term impact of psychiatric drugs on children and adolescents. An excellent PBS documentary is *The Medicated Child*.

While pharmaceutical firms actively promote psychiatric drugs to psychiatrists and the public, they rarely acknowledge the serious side effects these drugs can produce. While sometimes these side effects can be quite mild, such as a dry throat or feeling groggy, others can result in more severe problems. Weight gain is a common side effect of many antidepressants and can cause serious physical health problems as well as reinforcing a negative body image. Tardive dyskinesia is a Parkinson like physical response reflecting the way antipsychotics can interfere with muscle control. However, pharmaceutical companies have been quick to advertise for additional medications to combat tardive dyskinesia. Antidepressants are well known to cause mania and suicidal ideation, and Ritalin has also been found to produce drug induced psychosis (Whitaker, p. 237–8). What is needed is a careful and cautious use of medications after alternative nonmedical treatments have been implemented, especially with children and adolescents. Cognitive behavioral therapy, group or family therapy, open dialog therapy, and peer supports should all be part of an integrated model of treatment. However, therapeutic interventions are often not reimbursed by insurance, either private or public. Many mental health providers do not accept insurance, requiring patients to pay out of pocket. Even if affordable there is a clear lack of mental health care providers, as we have discussed. Consequently, there is an even greater reliance on psychiatric medications; the majority of the growth in mental health care expenditures has been for psychiatric medications. However, rather than advance nonmedical interventions, current reforms are based upon increasing mandatory care, or involuntary commitment, to "coerce" patients into taking their psychiatric medication.

Involuntary Treatment and Civil Commitment

Forced treatment is legally referred to as involuntary commitment which is court-ordered treatment to a hospital or to mental health treatment in an outpatient setting. Involuntary "civil" commitment is different from "criminal" commitment as no crime has been committed. Civil commitment can provide for court-ordered outpatient commitment, or mandatory community treatment. Hospitalization during the 1800s and early 1900s provided psychiatric treatment and care for those deemed mentally ill and most admissions were involuntary. Commitment was in the control of psychiatrists whose actions were assumed to be in the patient's best interest; all that was required was that the patient be mentally ill and that admission against the patient's will was necessary (Testa and West, 2010). By the mid-1900s, this view of benevolent care had come under attack as it became apparent that mental hospitalization often provided at best only custodial care, or at worst coercive control over deviant behavior. Standards for commitment moved from a medical, treatment model to a legal model. Legal restrictions were placed on commitment criteria, and debates continue today over the role of legal versus psychiatric criteria in determining who needs to be involuntarily committed and who does not.

The legal reforms of the 1960s and 1970s initiated due process protections to patients undergoing civil commitment, restricted involuntary commitment to those who were dangerous to themselves and/or others and limited the discretionary authority of psychiatrists. Another important limitation on the power to commit was the right of the patient to the least restrictive alternative. The constitutional basis for the least restrictive alternative is the idea that individuals have a right to freedom from unnecessary restraints. In practice, this meant that courts had to determine that patients were not being placed in a more restrictive environment than necessary. Outpatient commitment was developed as a middle road between involuntary hospitalization and community treatment by legally requiring an individual to go to the community mental health center for treatment, generally medication. A recurrent issue in understanding the impact of the least restrictive mandate as well as outpatient commitment is whether community placements and supports are indeed available.

Perhaps, the most contentious issue in the legal reforms of the 1970s is the interpretation of the "dangerousness" criteria for civil commitment. In O'Connor versus Donaldson, the US Supreme Court defined dangerousness as the legal justification for involuntary commitment. Dangerousness to self or others as the basis for involuntary commitment is a refutation of the medical model and its claim that individuals need to be committed in order to receive treatment (Stone, 1975). Psychiatrists in general have maintained that they can determine the best interest of the patient, and that patients are often not able to make appropriate decisions about their care or treatment. In contrast, legal scholars tend to focus on patient's rights, and argue that if treatment is coerced it cannot be effective. Both Mental Health America and the Bazelon Center for Mental Health Law have policy statements opposing involuntary commitment unless the individual is in imminent danger of significant harm and when no less restrictive alternative is available. Even in these cases, patients need to be afforded full procedural protections and should be found either legally incompetent or provide informed consent for mental health treatments. In contrast, the Treatment Advocacy Center and E. Fuller

Torrey continue to support and advocate for forced treatment if an individual refuses treatment, even if they are not dangerous. Miller and Hanson (2016) provided an excellent overview of the debates over involuntary commitment.

Another contentious legal debate has been whether patients have a right to refuse treatment. While few disagree that patients have a right to treatment, many have argued that refusal of treatment is a sign of the patient's incompetence and need for involuntary treatment, generally forcible administration of medication. Anosognosia is a medical term that refers to a person's refusal of treatment as a symptom of their illness in that they do not recognize they are sick and need treatment. Forced medication is consequently seen as in the patient's best interest. A 1989 case heard in California (Riese vs St. Mary's Hospital) found that while individuals can be forcibly medicated in an emergency situation, in nonemergency settings the individual must be found incompetent. If treatment cannot be forced, there is little justification for involuntary commitment, although involuntary outpatient commitment has been seen as a mechanism by which individuals can be coerced to receive treatment. A very good movie is "55 Steps," which portrays Hillary Swank as the lawyer who fought for Riese's right to refuse treatment. The movie also shows the trauma of coerced treatment as well as the need for community supports and acceptance of PSMH.

Currently, there have been increased calls to expand criteria for involuntary commitment (both inpatient and outpatient) and treatment, not just in the United States but worldwide. Data from 2008 to 2017 show that rates of involuntary commitment increased in 11 out of 18 countries (Rains et al., 2019) despite a clear lack of evidence that involuntary commitment is beneficial. While involuntary commitment can be justified in the case of dangerousness to self or others, it is very difficult to determine who is in fact both mentally ill and dangerous. This goes back to the inherent ambiguity surrounding diagnosis, but also in assessing who poses a threat. "While we might all agree that mentally unstable people should not have easy access to firearms, we don't have a way of defining who exactly, these mentally ill people are" (Miller and Hanson 2016, p. 217). Domestic violence is a clear predictor of dangerousness yet is not generally used to screen those who acquire guns.

In the United States, calls for enhanced involuntary commitment have been in response to the rash of mass shootings and violence as well as to increased homelessness in many cities.

In New York City, the mayor has advocated for lessening constraints on the abilities of first responders to forcibly take people for psychiatric evaluation and ultimately allow for easier access to involuntary commitment. California's governor has also expanded the use of court-ordered treatment for psychiatric medications. However, there are many good reasons why people do not want to take psychiatric medications, including weight gain, side effects such as tardive dyskinesia, a notable lack of energy, and even an enhanced risk for suicide. Medications do not work for everyone and should not be forced.

Psychiatrists view the ethical issues of involuntary commitment in terms of conflict between beneficence (acting in the patient's best interest) and respect for patient autonomy (Testa and West, 2010). The concern is that patients who are not dangerous and who refuse psychiatric treatment are not getting appropriate care, may further decompensate, lose valuable social supports, and even end up living on the streets or in jail. Consequently, violations of the patient's autonomy (i.e. involuntary commitment) is justified under the grounds of beneficence. However, there has been a long term trend toward the criminalization of the mentally ill and today far too many people with mental illnesses are receiving care in jails or prisons rather than in mental health facilities. Individuals with mental illness who do end up in jail or prison generally have committed minor offenses, often related to survival strategies. In response to the criminalization of the mentally ill, many are calling for stricter commitment criteria and an expanded role for mental institutions (see Early 2006 for an excellent account). However, researchers and advocates point to the failure of the mental health system and the lack of community-based services as the source of the problem, not commitment criteria.

The dearth of community supports is a central issue in outpatient commitment, originally designed as a viable least restrictive alternative to inpatient commitment. There are number of terms used in different counties and states, including compulsory community treatment or supervision with the contrast between the term "treatment" as opposed to "commitment" illustrating the continued conflict between medical as opposed to legal justifications for coercion. The compromise is a view of outpatient commitment or treatment as a benign or benevolent form of social control, which is referred to as "assisted" community treatment. Whether assisted, involuntary, or compulsory outpatient care is less restrictive than being in a hospital, but still potentially coercive. However, the coercion is seen as therapeutic rather than punitive.

There is wide variability in the uses of outpatient commitment, both globally and in the United States. Countries and states in the United States have diverse criteria and legal standards for involuntary commitment and the right to refuse treatment. While evidence of dangerousness to self or others is often included in the legal criteria for commitment, dangerousness can include medication noncompliance. In practical terms, outpatient commitment is used for individuals with a history of treatment noncompliance in the community. Unfortunately, there is a lack of publicly available data to track rates of involuntary commitments, so we do not know how well it works or for whom. Consequently, it is difficult to arrive at any consensus over the usefulness of involuntary commitment in providing necessary access to care and treatment to those in need, or to protecting society from potentially dangerous individuals. Community mental health providers that adhere to recovery models of care emphasize the role of self-directed treatment and choice. If some control is necessary for an individual with serious MHP, providers are more likely to exercise therapeutic social control and balance client autonomy with some coercion (Perry, Frieh, and Wright, 2018). However, as we saw in the proceeding chapter, adequately trained mental health providers and other community supports are often simply unavailable. Tweedy (2024) described a young black woman who came to the emergency room after taking too many aspirin (deemed suicidal) who he had to involuntarily commit to a state psychiatric hospital as she lacked insurance and could not be admitted to the smaller private hospital which had limited bed space. He found this to one of the most difficult decisions he had to make, and he references the research evidence that black people are less likely to receive outpatient care and more liked to be involuntarily committed.

What is interesting is how public perceptions and opinions have changed over the debate between more or less coercion for people with serious MHPs. Referred to as the Magna Carta of Mental health law, the Lanterman–Petris–Stout Act (LPS Act) was passed in the United States in 1967 and mandated that psychiatric treatment could only be forced if the patient was either dangerous or severely disabled. The LPS Act also called for enhanced voluntary community care and was used as a model by many jurisdictions and western societies. Barnard (2022) examined the public discourse surrounding the LPS Act as reflected in newspaper accounts, examining 575 articles over a 50 years' time period. He identified five major frames by which the public has viewed the policy debates over how to deal with the social problem of mental health (Box 12.1).

BOX 12.1 Public Discourse over Mental Health Reform

1960s: The Mental Health Revolution. An emphasis on the civil rights (civil liberty) of patients and restrictions on involuntary treatment in favor of voluntary community care.

1970s: Falling Through the Cracks. Concerns over the failure of community-based care due to the lack of resources and services, with board and care homes and single occupancy hotels providing those with serious MHPs a place to live. One psychiatrist in an article cited by Barnard raised concern about "abandoning kids liberating them before we have a chance to heal them."

1980s–1990s: Excessive Deinstitutionalization (DE). This period is critical of DE, and points to the rise in homelessness, trans institutionalization where PSMH were on the streets, or in nursing homes, or most tragically, in the criminal justice system. Barnard found that 90% of the statements used in the newspaper articles were by parents who wanted to see expanded civil commitment criteria for their children.

1990s–2000s. Dangerous Brain Diseases. In accordance with the Decade of the Brain, public discourse focused on MHPs as brain diseases which could (and should) be treated with psychiatric medications. Refusal of medication was seen as evidence of mental illness and that medications had to be forced. Without medication, PSMH could become dangerous to either themselves or others.

2010s: Re-institutionalizing those Dying in the Streets. This frame continued the concerns of the previous periods, but with an enhanced emphasis that involuntary commitment was justified to provide a safe place for people with SMHP.

The researchers found a notable lack in these public discourses that the failure of voluntary community-based care is a result of inadequate funding for community services. PSMH had (and still have) no place to go. Furthermore, even those with insurance face significant barriers to mental health treatment which can cost thousands of dollars for even short periods of care. However, many PSMH lack insurance. In the current "climate of opinion," PSMH are further demonized by the linkage of mass violence and shootings to MHPs. Another interesting observation is the voices that are missing from the newspaper accounts described by Barnard, patients and those living with severe MHPs. The interviews Miller and Hanson (2016) conducted show that people living with serious MHPs are highly critical of involuntary treatment and forced medication. What is also missing is any discussion of how community supports can be enhanced for meaningful recovery.

Criminalization

One of the justifications offered for enhanced involuntary mental health treatment is that far too many people with MHPs end up in the criminal justice system. Beginning in the 1970s, it had become apparent that prisons were replacing mental hospitals in a trend that looked similar to that of deinstitutionalization, where patients were moved from hospitals to the community. Now, we see that jails and prisons have replaced mental hospitals. However, it was not that patients who had once been in mental hospitals ended up in prisons, which would be a form of trans institutionalization. Instead, the lack of community-based mental health care led to growing number of individuals with MHPs having encounters with the criminal justice system. Prisons became the new asylums.

Hiday and Ray (2017) identified five subgroups of people with severe MHPs who end up in the criminal justice system. In order of frequency, the largest group are those who commit only minor misdemeanor nuisance crimes. These may include loitering or engaging in disturbing behavior such as talking to themselves (i.e. disturbing the peace). If they were not judged by police to be mentally ill they would probably not be arrested. The second group are those whose criminal offenses involve mostly survival behaviors, such as shoplifting, stealing food, pan-handling, or public indecencies (urinating in public). This second group of "offenders" are poor, often homeless, and simply lack the social supports to survive in the community. For both of these first two groups, jail diversion and mental health treatment is recommended, but if these programs are not available, jail becomes the only option.

The third group of people who end up in the criminal justice system are those with substance use problems; the substance use may have led to mental health issues, or the mental health issues may have led to substance use problems. These individuals may be under the influence and acting out. Public intoxication, a drug overdose, or drug induced psychosis all lead to encounters with law enforcement. The Opioid epidemic has certainly been driven by the mental health crisis and vice versa. However, treatment options for those with co-occurring behavior health problems are very limited, especially in rural and under-served communities.

The fourth group of offenders with mental health problems are those who have character disorders, such as antisocial personality disorder, and have high rates of violence against others. The fifth group is the smallest and includes the relatively few individuals who are delusional and whose delusions drive them to violence. However, these individuals certainly receive a great deal of attention and fit the public stereotype of a mass murderer or psychotic sociopath. These last two groups commit the kinds of crimes that are most closely associated with dangerousness. However, it is important to realize that very few people with MHPs in the community threaten or assault others, generally less than 20% using data from legal and medical records as well as patient self-report (Hiday and Ray, 2017). In fact, a person with a MHP is much more likely to be a victim of a crime or violence.

Once police are involved, people with MHPs are much more likely to be arrested, and are also more likely to be incarcerated. Often the obvious mental health problem led to a determination that an individual is "incompetent to stand trial" and they are then held in either the jail or prison or an available forensic mental health facility until they are judged competent to stand trial. Even a person with a severe MHP such as schizophrenia can be judged competent; the issue is whether their MHP prevents them from making a rational decision or acting in their own best interests. The end result is that many individuals spend a great deal of time incarcerated for MHPs while they are awaiting trial.

Criminalization also involves the reality that those who are found guilty serve longer sentences than individuals facing the same criminal offense but who have no previous MHPs. In addition, people with MHPs are more likely to be denied bail and parole. As the "new asylums" prisons can provide some level of mental health care, but the ability to do so and the quality of care varies widely. There are certainly accounts of proactive prisons who have worked to enhance their capacity to provide mental health care, and some awful facilities where mentally ill prisoners are stripped naked and placed in isolation (Early, 2006). However, while prisons can indeed provide "better" mental health care, they are clearly not the solution; instead, enhanced jail diversion programs and assertive community treatment are needed. Jails and prisons are not equipped to provide adequate mental health care; their primary purpose is control as well as punishment. The current shortage of those trained in mental health and willing to work in the criminal justice system will only lead to increased use of coercion or medication to control those with mental health problems. However, even if fortunate enough to be released from prison or jail, individuals with a criminal record will have a very hard time with what is referred to as "re-entry" – finding a place to live, a job, income, and mental health care.

Concluding Thoughts

MHPs are experienced at the individual level as a personal trouble. However, this is also a public issue or a social problem which affects society at large. Our current societal response is one of medicalization, forced treatment, and criminalization. Rather than provide meaningful community supports, we rely on the criminal justice system to warehouse those with serious MHPs and who are perceived to be a threat. It is clear that criminalization is a social "problem that represents the greatest scandal of our health care system, and a situation which should embarrass all thoughtful citizens" (Mechanic, 2006; p. 80). Tweedy (2024, p. 12) also lamented that "the all too frequent criminalization of mental health and drug-related problems speaks volumes about our society's fear, ignorance, and apathy toward those who suffer from them." Yet this situation has existed for over 40 years and indeed, has gotten only worse. Why aren't we embarrassed? The answer lies in the stigma of mental illness and our continued association of mental illness with common stereotypes and dangerousness. More fundamentally, we continue to view those who are marginalized by intersecting social statuses and mental illness as less than human.

Student Activities

Review any of the documentaries described below and identify some of the structural sources of criminalization. What needs to be done to reduce the criminalization?

1. The 2021 PBS Documentary *The Mysteries of Mental Illness* includes information on mental health treatment in the criminal justice system.

2. An earlier PBS Frontline *The New Asylums* (2005) examines a prison in OHIO which has implemented a separate system of care for prisoners with MHPs. While innovative and with a clear commitment to "better" mental health care, the video documents the realities of mental health treatment in prison. A follow-up documentary *The Released, 2009* examines the realities of "re-entry" by following some of the inmates who were released into the community and shows the many barriers they faced. The majority simply returned to the criminal justice system due to the lack of community supports.

3. A recent initiative with PBS Frontline and the Charlotte-based radio station (WFAE) resulted in a ten part series called "Fractured" which provides in-depth analysis of the problems those with MHPs face once they get involved with the Criminal Justice system. This series is now available as a podcast and as a PBS documentary.

References

Barnard, A. (2022). From the "magna carta" to "dying in the streets": media framing of mental health law in California. *Society and Mental Health* 12 (2):155–174.

Carlat, D. (2010). *Unhinged: The Trouble with Psychiatry – A Doctor's Revelations about a Profession in Crisis*. New York, NY: The Free Press.

Conrad, P. (2007). *The Medicalization of Society: On the Transformation of Human Conditions into Treatable Disorders*. Baltimore, MD: Johns Hopkins University Press.

Early, P. (2006). *Crazy: A Father's Search Through America's Mental Health Madness*. New York: G.P. Putnam.

Hiday, V. and Ray, B. (2017). Mental illness and the criminal justice system. In: *A Handbook for the Study of Mental Health*, 3e (ed. T.L Scheid and E.R Wright), 467–492. Cambridge: University Press.

Kolker, R. (2020). *Hidden Valley Road: Inside the Mind of an American Family*. New York: Anchor Books, a division of Penguin Random House, LLC.

Mechanic, D. (2006). *The Truth About Health Care: Why Reform Is Not Working in America*. New Brunswick, NJ: Rutgers University Press.

Miller, D. and Hanson, A. (2016). *Committed: The Battle Over Involuntary Psychiatric Care*. Baltimore, MD: Johns Hopkins University Press.

Perry, B.L., Frieh, E. and Wright, E.R. (2018). Therapeutic social control of people with serious mental illness: An empirical verification and extension of theory. *Society and Mental Health* 8 (2):108–122.

Rains, L.S., Zenina T., Dias M.C. et al. (2019). Variations in patterns of involuntary hospitalisation and in legal frameworks: An international comparative study. *Lancet Psychiatry* 6 (5):403–417.

Stone, A.A. (1975). *Mental Health and Law: A System in Transition.* DHEW Publication 76–176. Rockville, MD: National Institute for Mental Health, Center for Studies of Crime and Delinquency.

Testa, M. and West, S.G. (2010). Civil commitment in the United States. *Psychiatry* 7 (10):30–40.

Tweedy, D. (2024). *Facing the Unseen: The Struggle to Center Mental Health in Medicine.* New York: St. Martin's Press.

Whitaker, R. (2010). *Anatomy of an Epidemic: Magic Bullets, Psychiatric Drugs and the Astonishing Rise of Mental Illness in America.* New York, NY: Crown Publishers/Random House.

CONCLUSION

Vision for the Future: What Would a Mentally Healthy Society Look Like?

Where are we now? Community-based systems of care remain highly fragmented and underfunded. Instead of providing integrated community-based treatment, systems of mental health care have responded to wider institutional demands for cost containment. Beginning in the 1990s, both private and public systems of mental health care have moved to managed care models, with an emphasis on controlling costs and short-term treatment. The result has been increased reliance upon psychiatric medications to control the symptoms of mental health problems (MHPs), with less and less emphasis on therapy or rehabilitation. Mental health care has been medicalized with few individuals receiving the needed social supports for their social welfare needs to be addressed. The failure of community-based care has resulted in criminalization of those whose MHPs bring them into contact with the criminal justice system, which has become the de facto mental health system.

In addition, we face critical shortages of mental health care providers, especially those with the background and training to work in the criminal justice system. Increased use of peer supports and prosumers can help alleviate not only the shortage of professionally trained provides, but their burnout. Prosumers and volunteers can be educated via cross-training using materials developed by international and national agencies. Local level community expertise and the lived experience of consumers should be utilized to develop educational opportunities to identify and solve community gaps in services. Every community is different, and the types of services which can enhance recovery vary widely. Driven by local contexts, cross-training can both enable and empower individuals, families, and providers.

There is no one right template for cross-training, just as there is no one template for recovery. Instead, cross-training can assist providers and consumers to develop new solutions which can enhance local resources devoted to recovery. Cross-training enables both participants and the larger community and is an important mechanism in developing a collaborative community system of mental health care. In the United States, the Affordable Care Act included provisions for training and increased funding and supports for both mental health and cross-training; both of which should continue to be a national priority. The Biden administration has also extended supports for not only mental health care, but for training the mental health workforce. In September of 2024, the Biden–Harris administration earmarked 68.5 million in grants to support mental services provided by two key agencies. The Substance Abuse and Mental Health Administration can receive funding to address campus suicide prevention efforts and child traumatic health initiatives and the US Department of Health and Human Services will address infrastructure technology issues, including telehealth. Both agencies are critical to the collection of data on mental health needs and services.

The WHO 2022 *World Mental Health Report* also advocates for community-based mental health care, broadly defined as any care provided outside an institution. Community-based care must place people first and be accessible and integrate the diverse array of social supports and services necessary for mental health (WHO, 2022: section 7.1). For most countries, this will require a major restructuring of not only the mental health system, but primary health care and social services. The WHO prioritizes peer support services, psychosocial rehabilitation, supported living services, and greater opportunities for empowerment. In addition to changing involuntary commitment practices, they provide recommendations for promoting noncoercive practices. Service providers need to be educated and receive systematic training on the impact of power differences and learn noncoercive techniques which enhance communication and trust. Fundamentally, a dedicated community-based care system can protect human rights, reduce stigma, and provide for an enhanced quality of life. Developing a comprehensive community-based mental health system will involve planning and support from political leaders, public health agencies, healthcare providers, researchers, advocates, and those most directly impacted by MHPs.

The WHO 2022 World Mental Health Report provides numerous examples of successful efforts at reform. These include deinstitutionalization in Brazil (WHO, 2022: Box 7.2), the use of lay therapists in Uganda and Zambia to treat depression in women and adolescents (WHO, 2022: Box 7.4), the integration of mental health into primary health care settings in the Islamic Republic of Iran (WHO, 2022: Box 7.8). There is also an evidence-based protocol for guided self-help (Improving Access to Psychological Therapies) which was developed in the United Kingdom and has been used as a model in several other countries with research finding significant improvements in anxiety and depression (WHO, 2022: Box 7.6). Beyond these efforts to improve mental health care, the 2022 WHO report also details the need for enhanced mental health services in schools and the criminal justice system. Critical social services including child protection, education and training, opportunities for employment, and access to essential social benefits also need to be enhanced. Transforming mental health care for all will involve commitment as well as the willingness and ability to reshape existing systems of care. A final figure from the 2022 WHO World Mental Health Report articulates clearly the principles for what an ideal system of mental health care would look like, contrasting Before key shifts are implemented, with After transformation (WHO, 2022: Figure 8.2). These principles can be used by local communities to develop goals and benchmarks to guide advocacy and policy development.

We return to the four key sociological perspectives outlined in the introduction: social context, integration, stress, and stigma. As we have articulated throughout this book, our social structures (context) and our social relationships (integration) are all related to our experience of stress and MHPs. The stigma associated with MHPs then reduces our ability to provide adequate care or resources for the kinds of social transformations articulated by the 2022 WHO World Mental Health Report. A first step we can all make is to engage in efforts to reduce stigma, which involves labeling and marginalizing of those who are different. Definitions of normal and abnormal are defined within a given social context and can be changed. Efforts to reduce social inequality will not only change the social context but will reduce the differential effects of stress. Efforts to bring people together (integration) will also reduce stigma and provide needed community and social supports. There are many theoretical frameworks which address the embeddedness of individuals within societal organizations and larger system level frameworks, the most widely used being the social ecological model. In sociology, we often refer to the linkages of the micro (the individual level) to the meso (organizational level) to the macro (structural level). In our 2021 book, *Ties That Enable: Community Solidarity for People Living with Serious Mental Health* Problems, we developed the Wholistic Framework for Mental Health, which we have modified to address the persistence of stigma at the micro, meso, and macro levels (Figure 1).

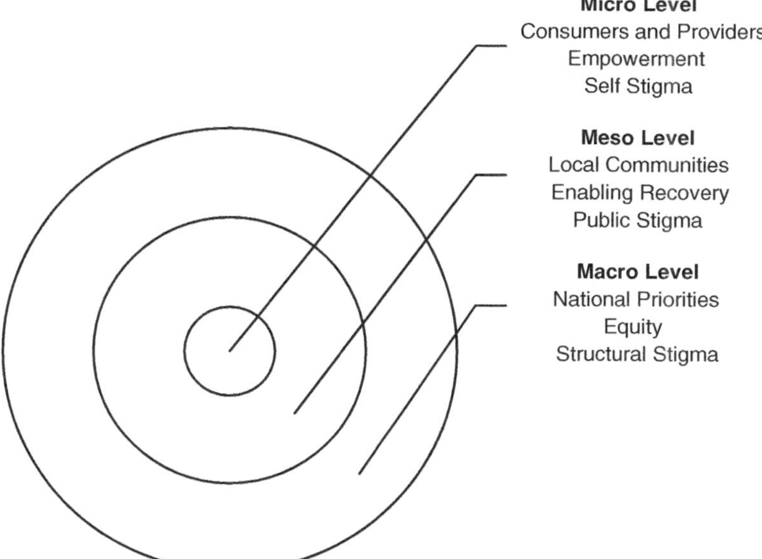

FIGURE 1   Wholistic Framework for Mental Health

Reforms must be both bottom up from the community with a priority on local level advocacy and provision of social supports to needy individuals, and top down from international and national bodies which can provide financing and standards for care. We need individuals (including consumers, prosumers, providers, and advocates) who are resilient and empowered to make meaningful changes. At the same time, communities need to provide adequate supports for recovery and opportunities for community engagement which empower individuals. However, the wider social and economic system constraints the opportunities available to both individuals and communities – that is, we operate within a system of pervasive social inequality which reinforces stigma and marginalization. At the systems level, we must work toward reforms that move the entire society to greater equity and social justice, which will then reduce the stigma associated with multiple forms of marginalization. We challenge readers of this book to identify ways that they can empower themselves and advocate for broader structural reform, and consequently reducing the impact of the mental health crisis on their communities.

Student Learning Activity

Access the World Health Organization's website and look for updates to their 2022 Report Mental Health Report as well as for global and community initiatives to address mental health. Where are we making progress and where have initiatives stalled? What factors are important to actual transformations to mental health? What vision do you see for mental health care in your community and what role can you play in making that happen?

Reference Cited

World Health Organization. 2022. *World Mental Health Report: Transforming Mental Health For All. World Mental Health Organization.*

Appendix A
Documentary to Accompany the Entire Course

The Mysteries of Mental Illness: Explore The Evolution in Understanding Mental Illness. 2021. WBGH Educational Foundation. A production of Pangloss Films for GBH Studio Six. Available through PBS. Summary provided by Dr. Scheid.

Part I Evil or Illness?

The documentary begins with the story of a woman boxing in the 2021 Olympics, dealing with her obsessive-compulsive disorder (OCD), and then goes to a black man with multiple diagnoses of bipolar, PTSD, anxiety. Citing lifetime prevalence rates, the video notes that half of all Americans are diagnosed with a mental illness. Mental health problems (MHPs) have increased due to COVID-19 and subsequent increased health inequities. Stigma is also addressed, and while we know more about the role of stigma, "less is being done" to address it.

Having introduced the contemporary face of mental health conditions, the series provides historical background and context, narrated by Andrew Scull (a noted historian and sociologist). The major point is that culture has shaped our perceptions of who is mentally ill and ideas about what is normal, asking "who fits in with cultural norms?" There is an overview of treatment of hysteria in women in late 1800s, and the role of religion. The documentary returns to stigma, with mental illness linked to morality, or views of appropriate normative roles and behaviors.

A woman experiencing suicidal thoughts laments that "I wasn't just losing my future ... I was losing my mind." What is the Mind? The video turns to John Locke and his views of the importance of thinking, and then the historic example of King George who was diagnosed as mentally ill even though he actually had a physical problem (an older movie but excellent is *The Madness of King George*). The video documents the horrific treatments of the 1700s, including bleeding and the use of leaches, and then moves to schizophrenia and schizoaffective disorder (schizophrenia with depression) – making the point that there is no "clinical pattern" to the behaviors associated with either.

The documentary turns to the work of Sigmund Freud, who initially sought biological roots to our thoughts and feelings, which was an application of Darwinian ideas. Freud made important distinctions between the unconscious and conscience, and between psychosis and neurosis. While Freud's ideas have been distorted, he did misunderstand early childhood development in terms of the Oedipal stages. Part I ends with a return to COVID and the mental health crisis, which points to vulnerabilities in our society.

Part II Who Is Normal?

Part II begins with the story of a trans Asian American person who felt "completely alone." The point being made is that there is no simple answer to who is, or is not, normal. The video addresses sociological ideas about the social origins of behavioral norms, deviance, and labeling theory. The historical context provided is the experience of being a black man during slavery. Whites labeled Blacks who wanted to run away as having a mental illness (referred to as drapetomania) which raises important questions about conformity and social control as well as the legacy of racism in our society.

Part III Rise and Fall of the Asylum

Continuing the points about racism in the previous segment, this episode starts with a Black man who is in jail (the new asylum) with 4–5 diverse diagnoses, which he thought were the result of his incarceration. Racism clearly plays a role, of the many who are incarcerated in the Cook County prison (Chicago), 40% have a diagnosis of mental illness and of that 40%, 90% are people of color. This points to institutionalized racism and treating behavioral issues as MHPs.

"After centuries of searching there are still no treatments... the only constant is stigma." The video makes the important point with historical evidence that those with mental health conditions were not viewed as fully human. Hospitals and prisons serve social control functions, protecting society from dangerous and deviant behavior with a blurred line between treatment and punishment.

Part III also provides an overview of Dorothea Dix and her promotion of "moral treatment" with a focus on self-control. While there was no national reform based on moral treatment, many states in the U.S. and some countries implemented a moral, therapeutic model of the asylum to provide a restful, "curative" environment with the goal of rehabilitation: "people need things to do of their own choice."

However, racism again played an important role with Jim Crow policies following the Civil War leading to enhanced social control of minorities and poor and marginalized people. Asylums became places where people were not only "out of mind, but also out of sight and forgotten." There is a good description of Pilgrim State on Long Island, which housed 13,000 patients and implemented a number of what can only be described as bizarre treatments, though with good intentions. The video moves to issues of sexual sterilization and eugenics in Nazi Germany.

New treatments increasingly focused on the Brain, with little understanding of the brain leading to radical treatments including lobotomy. In 1941, Rosemary Kennedy (who had been institutionalized for her promiscuous behavior as a young woman) was lobotomized, a procedure more often used for women to make them docile. Husbands were happy to see their wives content to do housework. In the 1950s, new drugs provided for "chemical lobotomies" – controlling behavior based on still unproven theories about a chemical imbalance in the brain.

The year 1963 brought the Community Mental Health Centers Act (CMHC) introduced by President John Kennedy which sought to relocate mental health care away from state institutions to community based care. There were also a variety of legal decisions mandating the "least restrictive alternative" that patients should not be forced into hospitals if they could survive in the community. However, funding never met the demand, a dilemma we experience to this day between the need for comprehensive, integrated systems of care and the costs of such care. Currently, 90% of the resources made available the 1963 CMHC Act are no longer available.

The 1980s brought Ronald Reagan's reforms to mental health, which block granted federal dollars to states to do as they wished. State hospitals retained their federal funding, but community-based care was severely undercut, leading to the criminal justice system becoming the "defacto" system of care. Blacks are still more likely to be incarcerated and diagnosed with a mental illness, though less likely to receive care. The Criminal Justice system can only provide medications (not therapy), but medications cannot be provided upon release leading to a viscous cycle. The third segment ends with a transition to Part IV, describing newer scientific advances which look at the role the environment plays on our biochemical systems, based on research on the intergenerational exposure to trauma.

Part IV New Frontiers

The final segment opens with a young white man with OCD who has struggled on a daily basis for eight years to control his breathing. He tried psychotherapy, medications, and cognitive behavioral therapy for his obsessive-compulsive behavior and is now "just biding my time for surgery." This segment introduces new advances in neuroscience, which views mental illness as arising in the brain, but is complicated by environmental and historical context. There is a good overview of the role played by diverse regions of the brain, with the frontal lobe (also targeted by lobotomy) and the basal grandia regions serving as controls for mental functions. Older ideas about different regions of the brain controlling behavior have been replaced by ideas about the connections between regions in the brain.

The OCD patient will undergo "Deep Brain Stimulation" to correct his "faulty wiring" in the brain. While not used much for OCD, the procedure has had some success in treating Parkinsons. The "Deep Brain Stimulation" worked for this patient, but involved three brain surgeries where electrodes were implanted into different regions of the brain, and a battery in the patient's chest that the patient and the physician can manipulate. The patient found "the compulsion completed gone" and the physician commented "hopefully he will feel more normal, more like himself." There is once again a great historical overview with videos of previous so called "treatments" which focused on the brain, including lobotomies, electric shock therapy (ECT), and insulin therapy which put the body into a state of shock.

ECT is very interesting and has been found to reduce mania as well as depression, but it does come at the cost of some memory loss. ECT reduces symptoms for those with long-term depression for whom nothing else has worked, including the elderly who face increased rates of depression associated with aging. However, we STILL do not know how, or why it works. As with insulin therapy, the idea is to produce a shock to the body, which is thought to "reboot the brain." Current use of ECT is very different than that depicted in the historical videos; muscle relaxers and lower doses of electricity are now used to avoid convulsions. Still, patients undergo numerous "treatments" which are not at all pleasant.

There is another segment on the use of psychedelics, dating back to the 1960s and outlawed as they were used by "hippies" to achieve a new awareness, but which also led to nonconforming behaviors. Today, psychedelics are again being used, with funding for research growing. MDMA, the basis for the feel good drug ecstasy, is in the final stages of FDA approval for PTSD. While MDMA does led to new insights about emotions, thoughts and feelings, we still do not know HOW these drugs work. Researchers think they operate by changing the patterns in our brains. The new frontier for neuroscience is finding the patterns in the brain and changing how diverse systems in the brain communicate with one another.

The segment ends with a good discussion of public distrust of psychiatry, and points to the structural problems of incarceration, racism, homelessness, and lack of access to care. Psychiatry needs to go to the community, and an example is given of "Barbershops for Black Men" – places where we receive social support and connections. In the African American Community, historic trauma and discrimination have been normalized.

Appendix B
Suggested Course Reading

Robert Kolker. 2021. *Hidden Valley Road: Inside the Mind of an American Family*. New York. Anchor Books. Summary provided by Dr. Scheid.

Introduction

Kolker is a journalist who was awarded a Guggenheim in 2011 for Criminal Justice Reporting. and his previous book *Lost Girls*, was one of NYT 100 most notable books. The data in *Hidden Valley Road* are based on hundreds of hours of interviews and access to the medical records of the family obtained in 2017 following the death of the mother. The information was made available by the youngest daughter (Lindsay, now in her 50s), who ultimately became involved in the care of her older brothers diagnosed with schizophrenia as they aged.

Hidden Valley Road is based on the story of the Galvin family but intertwines their story with a very readable history of the treatment (or lack) for those diagnosed with schizophrenia. The Galvin's (Don and Mimi) had 12 children; 10 boys followed by 2 girls after which Mimi was told having any more children was medically dangerous. Of the 10 boys, six developed severe mental health problems (MHPs), with diagnoses of schizophrenia and for one, bipolar disorder. All exhibited psychosis and had extensive contacts with the criminal justice and mental health systems. As noted in the preface (xvii), "One of the consequences of surviving schizophrenia for 50 years is that sooner or later, the cure becomes as damaging as the disease."

The other story in *Hidden Valley Road* is the history of the role of the NIMH and researchers who searched for genetic, neurological, and biochemical sources of schizophrenia. The book does an excellent job of addressing the major theories, treatments, and understandings of mental illness as well as a very readable review of the scholarship that is critical of psychiatric research. Kolker documents not only how treatment changed over time, but how the stigma of mental illness changed. While *Hidden Valley Road* is not written by a sociologist, it has important implications for understanding our culture's commitment to finding a "cure" or solution to schizophrenia. Kolker (p. 319) argued "Our culture looks at diseases as problems to solve... Too often, scientists get lost in their own silos, convinced their theory works to the exclusion of everyone else's." Just as with therapy, scientific progress is not always about breakthroughs and miracle cures, but gradual progress with many theories being abandoned when supporting evidence is lacking.

The Family Story

The book describes in detail the experiences of each of the children, focusing attention on the eldest, Donald, who had the most extensive contacts with the mental health system. Donald moved back and forth from home and various institutions until his placement in an assisted living facility where Lindsay visits him. Donald was briefly married and tried to kill himself and his wife; he had a history of suicide attempts and violence with his first signs of psychosis appearing in 1966. Jim, the second son, also receives a great deal of attention as he not only had psychotic episodes (dating to 1969), we learn he abused the two young girls and several of his younger brothers. He is married and the two girls often visited Jim and his wife to escape the chaos in the family with not only Donald, but the violence at home with eight competitive and combative brothers. The history of abuse comes out slowly and is not recognized until the girls are much older and out of the house.

Michael, the fifth son, also had many MHPs and encounters with both the criminal justice and mental health systems as he traveled around the country is a typical post hippie fashion. He spends time in California working with Brian, the fourth boy who had a promising career in music. Seemingly, out of the blue Brian shot his ex-girlfriend in the face and then himself. It turns out he had been prescribed an antipsychotic days before he died. This was a shock to the family who had to finally acknowledge there was a serious problem in the family. Matt and Joe also were diagnosed with schizophrenia. Peter, the last boy before the two girls were born, also developed MHPs and was institutionalized, though diagnosis and treatment point to bipolar rather than schizophrenia.

Nature versus Nurture

A major theme of the book is over the source, or etiology of serious mental illness, with a focus on schizophrenia. Since schizophrenia is "universal" with a relatively rare prevalence rate it is assumed there must be some specific mechanism, or cause. There is extensive research and scholarship on schizophrenia which all points to some degree of a biological or genetic role, as well as environmental features. The focus for much of the research has been on finding that internal source of schizophrenia. However, as Kolker noted in the preface (xx–xxi), "psychiatrists, neurobiologists, and geneticists all believed the code for the condition had to be there somewhere, but have not been able to locate it." Kolker begins with a short history of schizophrenia, going back to King Henry and Bleuler who coined the term. Bleuler did not mean a split personality by the term, schizo, but a split between the inner world of the individual (who is hearing voices, and experiences delusions and hallucinations) and the outer world: that is between perception and reality. He reviews the insights of Freud, Jung, Lacan, and Foucalt, noting areas of contention.

Kolker provides a consideration of the Galvin family environment, telling the story of the younger years and relationship between the parents, Don and Mimi. In 1980, the NIMH began studying the Galvins, as did ultimately the University of Colorado Health Sciences Center, and in later years pharmaceutical companies. Don and Mimi are certainly outliers in having 12 children, and Mimi had to be strongly forbidden to have more children by her doctors. In addition, they shared an early commitment to falconry and learned how to tame and control these wild birds in much the same way as they later did with their children. Don completed his PhD at the age of 40 and the only picture of the entire family is at his commencement. He had lots of interests outside the home, including work with leading artists which was funded by the National Endowment of the Arts which drew him often to Santa Fe with residencies, concerts, and fundraisers. Later, in the book, we learn that he had affairs and was called Romeo by his friends. He also received Electric Shock Therapy for depression, something no one knew until Lindsay gained access to the hospital records.

Mimi, his wife, shared his passion for falconry and the arts, and often accompanied him to Santa Fe, though this dropped off significantly with more children, and then more children with serious MHPs. In many ways, she fits the prototype of the "schizophrenogenic" mother, and Peter's University therapist blamed her directly for Peter's problems. Noteworthy is that despite frequent calls of police to the house and hospitalizations of the boys with MHPs, Don and Mimi keep as much as they could hidden, reflecting both the private and public stigma of MHPs. Even when confronted by her two girls with the abuse suffered by them from brother Jim, Mimi defended Jim and then pointed to her own abuse when she was young.

There is evidence in the family history for the diathesis-stress hypothesis, that there is a biological threshold with environmental stressors triggering a psychotic episode. For example, when Brian's girlfriend broke up with him or when Donald's wife left him. An update to the diathesis-stress hypothesis is the vulnerability hypothesis, articulated by Robert Freedman in 1977. Genetic triggers could make the brain more vulnerable to environmental stressors and is often seen in hypersensitivity disorder where sounds and light create sensory disorders (such as seen in John Nash). Freedman developed a way to measure the reactions to lights and sounds; he found individuals with schizophrenia are overly sensitive to stimuli, but no genetic source has been found to account for this vulnerability. Currently, epigenetics continues to argue that certain genes are activated by the environment. Freedman has found a gene that is associated with schizophrenia, the CHANA gene which is linked to a receptor, which is also associated with nicotine. Individuals with schizophrenia have fewer of these receptors, and nicotine helps activate these receptors, helping individuals to focus outwardly. Another researcher (DeLisa) who had genetic data from the Galvin family found a genetic mutation shared by the brothers, SHANK2, which was not a cause of schizophrenia, but a potential mechanism. While a genetic source has not been found, studies of the physical brain pointed to anomalies. CT scans found damaged ventricles in the brains of individuals with schizophrenia. Likewise, brain researchers have found that the hippocampus region of the brain is smaller with those diagnosed with schizophrenia. However, there is no way to determine if the damage preceded the onset of schizophrenia or was caused by it.

Current understanding of schizophrenia builds upon the insights of Thomas Insel in 2010 (when he was Director of the NIMH) that it is not a disease, but a symptom that the brain is not working well; due to "a collection of neurodevelopmental disorders" (p. 272). Accordingly, the emphasis is shifting to prevention with some evidence that prenatal vitamins might prevent what "onset" of schizophrenia. However, the NIMH only spends 4.3 million on fetal prevention, despite evidence that half of all young school shooters had symptoms of developing schizophrenia.

Treatment

There are two primary forms of treatment for MHPs: medication and therapy. Ideally, both should be used and this is now the standard of care, but the emphasis has always been on medications. Deinstitutionalization is often associated with the development and availability of anti-psychotic drugs, and Thorazine was used in both inpatient and outpatient settings to control patients. Kolker notes that "even today no one knows for sure why Thorazine and other neuroleptic drugs do what they do" (p. 87). The dopamine hypothesis has been offered, hypothesizing that the drugs affect dopamine levels. However, Thorazine decreases dopamine and a newer drug which is very successful with some patients, Clozapine, increases dopamine. Some attention is also paid to the SSRIs, but neuroleptic drugs are still commonly used for schizophrenia. However, these drugs have negative consequences with long-term use. Jim and Joe both died of heart failure linked to long-term use of neuroleptics.

None of the boys were ever offered therapy. Peter (with bipolar) disease did not do well on drugs, and finally was offered Electroshock Therapy and after several weeks of treatment was declared symptom free. Lindsay did undergo extensive therapy, and her experience debunks the widely held assumption of a psychological breakthrough to deal with years living in an abusive environment. Lindsay had 25 years of intensive counseling to make sense of her life, despite her obvious resiliency her whole life. She ends up caring for her mother as she ages (and her mother was not easy) as well as the boys, providing them with tangible and emotional supports. Lindsay shows that we are not only a product of our genes, but of those who surround us, that "we are human because the people around us make us more human." One grandson, Jack, is enrolled into an extensive intervention program when he began exhibiting anxiety (due to a realistic fear of becoming mentally ill himself). He was able to resume school after several months. A nice ending to the family saga is that Kate, Lindsay's daughter, is working in a lab with Freedman as an undergraduate premed student.

Index

Printed and bound by CPI Group (UK) Ltd, Croydon, CR0 4YY

07/07/2026

14916222-0001